Rural Women's Health

Mental, Behavioral, and Physical Issues

Rural Women's Health

Mental, Behavioral, and Physical Issues

Editors

Raymond T. Coward, PhD
Lisa A. Davis, MHA
Carol H. Gold, PhD
Helen Smiciklas-Wright, PhD
Luanne E. Thorndyke, MD
Fred W. Vondracek, PhD

SPRINGER PUBLISHING COMPANY

Springer Publishing Company, Inc.
11 West 42nd Street
New York, NY 10036

Acquisitions Editor: Helvi Gold
Production Editor: Janice Stangel
Cover design by Joanne Honigman
Typeset by International Graphic Services, Inc., Newtown, PA

06 07 08 09 10 / 5 4 3 2 1

Library of Congress Cataloging-in-Publication Data

Rural women's health : mental, behavioral, and physical issues / editors Raymond T. Coward . . . [et al.].
    p. ; cm.
  Includes bibliographical references and index.
  ISBN 0-8261-2945-5
    1. Rural women—Health and hygiene—United States. 2. Rural women—Medical care—United States. [DNLM: 1. Rural Health.
  2. Women's Health. 3. Patient Acceptance of Health Care.
  4. Socioeconomic Factors. WA 309 R948 2006] I. Coward, Raymond T.
RA771.6.U6R87 2005
362.1'04257'0820973—dc22   2005022433

Printed in the United States of America by Sheridan Books, Inc.

Raymond T. Coward, MSW, PhD, is the Raymond E. and Erin Stuart Schultz Professor and Dean of the College of Health and Human Development at The Pennsylvania State University and is a professor of health policy and administration. His primary research interests are patterns of health and health care utilization among vulnerable populations, especially minority elders and residents of small towns and rural communities. Dr. Coward was the founding editor of *The Journal of Rural Health* (1985–1990), now in its 20th year of publication, and is the author or editor of eight books, including several focused on rural populations: *The Family in Rural Society* (1981), *Family Services: Issues and Opportunities in Contemporary Rural America* (1983), *The Elderly in Rural Society* (1985), *Health Services for Rural Elders* (1994) and *Aging in Rural Settings: Life Circumstances and Distinctive Features* (1998). He has also authored more than 125 journal articles and book chapters in the fields of gerontology, family studies, and health services research. In April 1996, Dr. Coward was awarded the *Professional Leadership Award* from the National Council on Aging. He has also been the recipient of the *Distinguished Academic Gerontologist Award* from the Southern Gerontological Society (1994) and the *Distinguished Researcher Award* from the National Rural Health Association (1993). In April 1991, Dr. Coward was named a *Distinguished Alumni* of Purdue University and in May 1991 he received the *President's Award* from the National Rural Health Association for his contributions to that professional association. In 1989 he was named the John K. Friesen Endowed Lecturer in Gerontology at Simon Fraser University (British Columbia) and in 1981 Dr. Coward received the *Distinguished Research Award* from the American Rural Health Association. He is a member of the honor societies of Phi Kappa Phi and Sigma Xi, and has been elected to *Who's Who in Science, Contemporary Authors* and *Outstanding Young Men of America*.

Lisa A. Davis, MHA, is the Director of the Pennsylvania Office of Rural Health, where she is responsible for the overall direction and leadership of the state office of rural health, including developing and sustaining linkages with state and national partners and expanding the office's role in enhancing the health status of rural Pennsylvanians. She is the immediate Past-President of the Pennsylvania Rural Health Association and immediate Past-Secretary of the

National Organization of State Offices of Rural Health's Board of Directors. She sits on the advisory boards of a wide range of national and statewide organizations and agencies, including the Board of Directors of Family Health Council of Central Pennsylvania, the Advisory Board of the Center for Rural Health Practice at the University of Pittsburgh at Bradford, and the Pennsylvania Rural Development Council. In addition to rural health issues, her special areas of interest focus on public health policy, women's health, special populations, and the un- and underinsured. Ms. Davis received the *2003 Outstanding Leadership Award* from the Pennsylvania Rural Health Association, the *2003 Distinguished Service Award* from the National Organization of State Offices of Rural Health, and the *2001 Award for Contributions to Public Health* from the Pennsylvania Public Health Association. Ms. Davis holds an undergraduate degree in Sociology/Psychology from Clarion University of Pennsylvania and a Master's in Health Administration from The Pennsylvania State University.

Carol Hancock Gold, PhD, is a faculty member in the Department of Biobehavioral Health, Penn State University, and an Associate Professor in the Institute of Gerontology at Jönköping University College of Health Sciences in Jönköping, Sweden. She received her Master's from Duke University and her Doctorate from The Pennsylvania State University. Dr. Gold's research focuses on gender differences in aging and health, and on the relationship between health-related quality of life and the use and misuse of prescription drugs. She has a special interest in women's health issues. Dr. Gold is also involved in a community-based volunteer health clinic.

Helen Smiciklas-Wright, PhD, is Professor of Nutrition and Director of the Diet Assessment Center in the Department of Nutritional Sciences at The Pennsylvania State University. Her research interests are in assessment of older adults who are at nutritional risk and the antecedents and consequences of risk. Research on nutrition screening and assessment has been conducted primarily with the Geisinger Rural Aging Study (GRAS). This is a cohort study of approximately 21,000 rural older Pennsylvanians. GRAS participants completed baseline nutrition and health screenings between 1994 and 1999. Wave 1 and 2 follow-up screenings have been concluded with the cohort, as have comprehensive nutritional studies of subsets of the population. Dr. Wright was co-editor with Drs. Gueldner and Burke of *Preventing and Managing Osteoporosis* (Springer Publishing, New York, 2000).

Luanne E. Thorndyke, MD, FACP, is the Associate Dean for Professional Development and Associate Professor of Medicine of The Pennsylvania State University College of Medicine. She is responsible for leading activities to recruit, sustain, and retain faculty, and for post-graduate educational programming for physicians, nurses, and allied health personnel. Initially serving as the Assistant Dean of Continuing Education at the College of Medicine, she has extensive experience in educational planning, program implementation, and accreditation standards. As a young physician and medical entrepreneur, she established a community-based private practice in Philadelphia. Advancing to clinical administration, she has served as the medical director of a large, inner-city public health clinic, an outpatient academic group practice, and as a board officer of a multihospital system. A board certified internist with certification in geriatrics and menopausal medicine, Dr. Thorndyke remains an active and established clinician with a primary focus in women's health and geriatrics. Dr. Thorndyke facilitates initiatives in women's leadership development and gender equity at The Pennsylvania State University College of Medicine. Born and raised in rural Nebraska, she is committed to improving the health and status of women and men, both rural and urban, through clinical practice, educational programs, administrative leadership, and community service.

Fred W. Vondracek, PhD, is Associate Dean for Undergraduate Studies and Outreach in the College of Health and Human Development at The Pennsylvania State University, Professor of Human Development in the Department of Human Development and Family Studies, and Honorary professor at the Friedrich Schiller University of Jena in Germany. Dr. Vondracek received his Doctorate in Clinical Psychology from Penn State University in 1968. His work has been published in numerous professional journals and books, and he has lectured both nationally and internationally on his developmental-contextual model of career development across the lifespan.

Contents

Contributors

Frank M. Ahern, PhD, is a faculty member in the Department of Bio-behavioral Health at The Pennsylvania State University, and the Director of the Medicine, Health, and Aging Project. He is also the Professor-in-Charge of the undergraduate program in Biobehavioral Health. Dr. Ahern received his master's and doctorate in Psychology from the University of Hawaii. Dr. Ahern currently directs a program of research related to pharmaceutical use among the elderly, healthy outcomes associated with use and misuse of pharmaceuticals, and evaluation of programs designed to reduce the risks of adverse drug-related outcomes.

Elizabeth G. Baxley, MD, is Professor and Chair of the Department of Family and Preventive Medicine at the University of South Carolina School of Medicine. She completed her family medicine training in 1987 at the Anderson Family Practice Residency Program, and then completed a faculty development fellowship at the University of North Carolina at Chapel Hill. She has served as a faculty member at the Anderson residency program, and has also been on faculty at Indiana University before returning to USC in 1994. At the USC School of Medicine she has served as Residency Program Director for Family Medicine and as Director of Faculty Development for the School of Medicine prior to becoming Chair in 2003. Her research interests are in women's health, health disparities, and medical education. She has been an investigator with the University of South Carolina's Rural Health Research Center for the past four years.

Jane Nelson Bolin, RN, JD, PhD, is an Assistant Professor of Health Policy and Management in the Texas A&M University's School of Rural Public Health. Dr. Bolin earned a Bachelor of Science in Nursing in 1978 (OHSU) and a Juris Doctor in 1982 from the University of Oregon. She practiced medical and employment related law for 13 years before leaving to earn her doctorate at The Pennsylvania State University. Dr. Bolin teaches Health Law and Ethics and Human Resources Management at Texas A&M School of Rural Public Health. Her current research includes Chronic Disease Management in Rural Areas (funded by HRSA and SWRHRC), Rural HIV/AIDS Prevention and Treatment, Health-Related QOL changes in patients after revascularization, and using forensic science to identify mistreatment deaths in long-term care facilities.

Caron Bove, PhD, MD, is a Research Associate in the Division of Nutritional Sciences at Cornell University. She is currently studying the interrelationships among food security, health, and body weight in rural low-income women, and body-weight changes of newlyweds. Her earlier work involved the qualitative study of the infant feeding decisions of low-income women, postpartum weight retention, and dietary changes of newlyweds. She holds a PhD in Nutrition from Cornell University and an MD from the University of Vermont.

Zoran Bursac, MPH, PhD, is Assistant Professor in the Department of Biostatistics, University of Arkansas for Medical Sciences. He completed his graduate work in biostatistics at the University of Oklahoma Health Sciences Center. He worked as a biostatistician for four years at the Oklahoma State Department of Health and his primary involvement was with the Oklahoma REACH 2010 project. He published several articles in peer-reviewed journals as the author or co-author, and has co-authored two book chapters. His main research interests include longitudinal data analysis, mixed models, missing data issues and statistical simulation and computing. Dr. Bursac is a member of the American Statistical Association.

Janis Campbell, PhD, is the Surveillance Coordinator for Chronic Disease at the Oklahoma State Department of Health. She has served in that position for four years. She has over 10 years experience with public health research and surveillance in Oklahoma. Dr. Campbell is the principal investigator for the Oklahoma Central Cancer Registry and the Oklahoma REACH 2010 Native American Project to Address Cardiovascular Disease and Diabetes. Dr. Campbell received her PhD in Anthropology in 1997 from the University of Oklahoma. Dr. Campbell is an adjunct faculty member at the Oklahoma University College of Public Health. She has published and presented locally and nationally on many occasions on topics related to health care among Native Americans in Oklahoma.

Gary A. Chase, PhD, is Professor in the Division of Biostatistics, Department of Health Evaluation Sciences at Penn State College of Medicine. He received a Bachelor of Arts magna cum laude from Harvard in 1966 and a PhD in Genetic Statistics from Johns Hopkins University in 1970. He served on the faculty at Johns Hopkins for 24 years, attaining the rank of professor in 1985. Subsequently he was appointed chief statistician at Georgetown University Medical Center and later at Henry Ford Hospital, prior to his appointment at The Pennsylvania State University in 2003. He served in an advisory capacity for both military and civilian sectors of the United States Government from 1972 to 2004 and was acting chief statistician of the Armed Forces Institute of Pathology from 1984 to 1985. He has published over 150 papers in refereed journals and is co-author of the widely cited text *Principles of Genetic Counseling*. His special interests include vital statistics, genetic risk prediction and statistical methods in genetic counseling.

Peggye Dilworth-Anderson, PhD, is a Professor at the School of Public Health in the Department of Health Policy and Administration, and is Director of the Center for Aging and Diversity at the Institute on Aging at the University of North Carolina-Chapel Hill. She received her Doctorate and Master's in Sociology from Northwestern University in sociology in 1972 and 1975, respectively. She received post-graduate training from the Midwest Council on Social Research at the University of Kansas in 1976–78, and other specialized training in Alzheimer's disease research at the Harvard Geriatric Education Center in 1985. Her areas of expertise include minority aging, family caregiving, intergenerational relations, and health disparities. She has received numerous awards and honors for her research that has been published in peer-reviewed journals and invited book chapters, in addition to being featured in *The New York Times, USA Today, The Christian Science Monitor* and other national and local newspapers.

Dr. Dilworth-Anderson has served in a number of leadership roles in the field of aging. She is currently chair of the behavioral and social science section of the Gerontological Society of America, and is also serving on the board of directors of the National Board of the Alzheimer's Association. She has served on two review panels for the National Institutes of Health, National Institute on Aging. Her professional affiliations include the American Sociological Association, the Gerontological Society of America, the American Public Health Association, and the National Council on Family Relations.

Kelli L. Dominick, PhD, is a Research Health Scientist at the Center for Health Sciences Research in Primary Care and the Epidemiologic Research and Information Center at the Durham, Virginia Medical Center, and is an Assistant Research Professor in the Department of Medicine at Duke University Medical Center. Dr. Dominick's research is focused on pharmacoepidemiology among older adults and the treatment of osteoarthritis. She is particularly interested in interventions that enhance quality of care for osteoarthritis in the primary care setting. Dr. Dominick is also trained as an exercise physiologist and is interested in the implementation of home-based physical activity programs among older adults with arthritis.

Sarah Gehlert, PhD, is an Associate Professor at the School of Social Service Administration of the University of Chicago, where she serves as Deputy Dean for Research, and the University's Institute for Mind and Biology. Dr. Gehlert is the Director of the NIH-funded University of Chicago Center for Interdisciplinary Health Disparities Research. She is Vice President of the Society for Social Work and Research and serves as Consulting Editor of *Social Work Research*, and on the Internal Review Board of *Social Service Research*. Dr. Gehlert was for eight years a social worker at the University of Missouri Hospitals in Columbia, Missouri.

Paula Goodwin, PhD, is currently a postdoctoral fellow with the Carolina Program in Healthcare and Aging Research of the University of North Carolina's Institute on Aging. She received her Bachelor's degree in Psychology (minoring in Sociology) from Wake Forest University in 1992. She received both her Master's and Doctorate in Human Development and Family Studies at the University of North Carolina at Greensboro in 1998 and 2001, respectively. In 2003, she completed a two-year fellowship with the Family Research Consortium III at the University of California-Los Angeles, and the University of North Carolina at Chapel Hill focusing on family processes and child/adolescent mental health in diverse contexts. Dr. Goodwin's major research interest is women's family roles and health outcomes, with an emphasis on race, geographic location, and household structure. Her work has appeared in the *Journal of Marriage and the Family* and in *Aging and Mental Health*.

S. Ann Hartlage, PhD, is an Assistant Professor in the Department of Psychiatry and Psychology at Rush University Medical Center and Rush Medical College. She is the winner of a *National Award for Research on*

Schizophrenia and Depression (NARSAD) Young Investigator Award. Dr. Hartlage has conducted research on depression in women, premenstrual dysphoric disorder (PMDD), and premenstrual exacerbation of other psychiatric disorders for the past eleven years. Prior to receiving her PhD, Dr. Hartlage taught adolescent inpatients in a psychiatric hospital and supervised classes for behaviorally disordered youth.

Debra A. Heller, PhD, is a Pharmacy Research Scientist for First Health Services Corporation and the Pennsylvania Pharmaceutical Assistance Contract for the Elderly (PACE). She is also an adjunct faculty member in the Department of Biobehavioral Health at Penn State University. Dr. Heller received a Master's and Doctorate in Genetics from The Pennsylvania State University. Her research interests include pharmaco-epidemiology, gerontology, and program evaluation. Dr. Heller is especially interested in the use of administrative claims-based databases to examine health outcomes and to evaluate public program efficacy.

Marianne Hillemeier, PhD, MPH, is an assistant professor in the Department of Health Policy and Administration at The Pennsylvania State University. She has multidisciplinary training in maternal and child health, with a Master of Science in Pediatric Nursing and certification as a Pediatric Nurse Practitioner, a Master of Public Health in Maternal Child Health, and a Doctorate in Sociology/Demography. She has published research related to trends and mechanisms underlying mortality differentials among children, and also related to disparities in women's health and fertility patterns and the implications of those disparities for child health outcomes. She is Director of the Research Core within the Central Pennsylvania Center of Excellence for Research on Pregnancy Outcomes, and is Co-Principal Investigator of the CePAWHS project. She is also conducting research on disparities in children's use of mental health services, on disparities in children's eligibility and enrollment in public health insurance, and on rural/urban differences in childhood asthma burden and school-based services.

Denise Jameson, MSN, is the Director of Community Health Education and Resources (CHER) since 1991. CHER provides education to the Inland Northwest and represents the four medical centers in Spokane, Washington. She holds a Bachelor of Science in Nursing from Gonzaga University and a Master's of Nursing from Whitworth College. Denise was the Diabetes Clinical Nurse Specialist and Diabetes Case Manager at Sacred Heart Medical Center from 1991 to 1999. She served as a missionary in Colombia, South America, from 1989 to 1991. She has worked in the health care field for over 30 years and believes that providing education to clients allows them to maintain optimum health.

Kelly Kovac, MA, is a NIMH predoctoral fellow at the University of Wisconsin-Madison School of Social Work. Her work is supported by a predoctoral training grant entitled "Research Training on Families and Mental Health Services." Kovac received her Master's in Social Work from the University of Chicago.

Warren Lambert, MA, completed this work while he was a graduate student at Marshall University working on his Master's in Clinical Psychology. He now teaches psychology at Somerset Community College in Kentucky, and he plans to pursue his doctorate in the future. Warren became interested in psychology while he was an undergraduate student at Ohio University. His current research interests include rural behavioral health and disorders of childhood.

Kathleen M. McNamara, PhD, ABPP, has provided psychological services to rural populations for over 25 years. She has been actively involved in advocacy and public policy formulation related to psychological services. As a member of the Board of Directors of the American Psychological Association (APA), Chairperson of the Committee on Rural Health, and in other leadership roles, she has served as a champion for rural issues and the unique needs of rural and frontier women. As a practitioner and trainer of professional psychologists entering rural practice, she is quite aware of rural health-care delivery problems, social and public policy issues which must be addressed to improve the quality of health care for rural residents, and the need for innovations in technology applications for both training and health-care delivery in rural areas.

Charity G. Moore, MSPH, PhD, completed the Master of Science in Public Health and a Doctorate in Biostatistics in 1997 and 2000 at the School of Public Health of the University of South Carolina (USC). After graduating, she worked in Chicago as Assistant Professor at Rush-Presbyterian-St. Luke's Medical Center in the Section of Biostatistics. In January 2002, she returned to the Arnold School of Public Health at USC as a Research Assistant Professor of Biostatistics in the Department of Epidemiology and Biostatistics. Dr. Moore is currently the Deputy

Director for the South Carolina Rural Health Research Center. Her research interests include analysis of complex sample survey data, mixed models, methods of handling missing data, and count data models.

Pamela L. Mulder, PhD, is an associate professor and the Director of the Institute for Rural Community Psychology at Marshall University in Huntington, West Virginia. She is the supervising editor of the *Journal of Rural Community Psychology*. Dr. Mulder obtained her doctoral degree in clinical psychology at the California School of Professional Psychology in Fresno, California in 1991. Her research interests are focused on issues related to interventions appropriate for rural communities and on factors that facilitate the development of resilience and wellness in rural residents.

Christine M. Olson, PhD, is the Hazel E. Reed Human Ecology Extension Professor of Family Policy in the Division of Nutritional Sciences at Cornell University. She received a Bachelor of Science in Experimental Foods in 1970 and a Master's and Doctorate in Nutritional Sciences in 1972 and 1974, respectively, from the University of Wisconsin-Madison. She joined the faculty of the Division of Nutritional Sciences at Cornell University as an Assistant Professor in 1975.

The nutritional concerns of women, infants, and children are the focus of Professor Olson's scholarly work. Presently, she is studying how recommendations for weight gain during pregnancy and health behaviors (eating, physical activity, and breastfeeding) relate to the development of obesity. Her group is following low-income, rural families over three years to study changes in their hunger and food insecurity status.

Cathy Parrett, DNSc, RN, received the Associate of Arts in Nursing and the Bachelor of Science degrees from the University of Tennessee-Martin, the Master of Science degree in Nursing from the University of Tennessee-Knoxville, with a concentration in Adult Health, and the DNSc from the University of Tennessee Health Sciences Center in Memphis. Dr. Parrett has several years of experience in nursing administration, clinical practice, and nursing education. She is actively involved in local and state nursing organizations. She is currently an Associate Professor of Nursing, teaching in the areas of nursing administration, and leadership and management in nursing. In addition, Dr. Parrett continues to work with older adults through health promotion and wellness activities.

Lisa Perkins, MS, a member of the Cherokee Nation, is the Director of Health Promotion for Cherokee Nation Health Services. Lisa holds a master's from Northeastern State University in College Teaching with an emphasis in Health. Lisa has been with the Cherokee Nation since 1991 and currently works closely with the Oklahoma State Department of Health Chronic Disease Division REACH 2010 Project and the Cherokee Nation Diabetes Program, and she chairs the Cherokee Nation Community Health Services Committee.

Janice C. Probst, PhD, is an Associate Professor in the Department of Health Services Policy and Management, Arnold School of Public Health at the University of South Carolina, and is Director of the South Carolina Rural Health Research Center. Dr. Probst's research focuses on health services issues important to rural populations, with an emphasis on communicating results to policy audiences. Her work has included national analyses using the complex data sets generated by the National Center for Health Statistics, such as the National Health Interview Survey and the National Ambulatory Medical Care Survey, analyses of patient data from billing data sets, and county level analyses. In 2001, Dr. Probst received the South Carolina Rural Health Association's *Researcher of the Year Award*.

Megan Romer, MS, is a research assistant in the Clinical Trials Coordination Center at the University of Rochester, where she provides statistical support and SAS programming for Parkinson's and Huntington's disease studies. She received her Master of Science in Statistics from The Pennsylvania State University in 2002. While at Penn State, Ms. Romer worked as a Senior Research Support Associate in the Department of Health Evaluation Sciences at the university's Hershey Medical Center. Her work focused primarily on geographic information systems to study the effects of air pollution on cardiovascular disease. She also did SAS programming for two major studies focused on the effects of living in a rural area, including the adverse pregnancy study, and numerous other projects. Ms. Romer received her Bachelor of Science from the State University of New York-Oswego in 2000 with a double major in Applied Mathematics and Applied Mathematical Economics and a minor in Statistics.

Judith A. Shinogle, PhD, is an Assistant Professor of Health Economics in the Clinical Pharmacy and Outcomes Sciences Department of the University of South Carolina. She has a joint appointment at the Arnold School of Public Health in the Health Services, Policy and Management Department and serves as faculty for the USC's Prevention Research Center. Dr. Shinogle received her Doctorate in Health Economics from

The Johns Hopkins University and was a National Institute of Mental Health Pre-Doctoral Fellow in Mental Health Economics. She has received the NCHS/Academy Health Policy Fellowship to study generosity of health and mental health insurance coverage. Her previous research has focused on private disability insurance, disability management, as well as mental health benefits. Her current research focuses on pharmacy benefit issues and economics of health care decision making. Her research on behavioral health care focuses on the effect of economic incentives on lifestyle changes such as smoking, substance abuse, physical activity, and obesity. Dr. Shinogle has published in *The Milbank Quarterly*, *Health Care Financing Review*, *Psychiatric Services*, and *Journal of Behavioral Health Services Research*. She has presented her work at various conferences including the Southern Economic Association, the Eastern Economic Association, and the Academy Health and International Health Economics Association.

In Han Song, MSW, is a Doctoral candidate at the School of Social Service Administration of the University of Chicago. His research interests are in culture and mental health and his dissertation topic is "Cross-Cultural Aspects of Premenstrual Dysphoric Disorder." He has a Bachelor of Arts from Yonsei University in Seoul, Korea, and a Master of Social Work from Washington University in St. Louis. He was a psychiatric social worker in Korea and is currently establishing the Korean-American Women's Mental Health Centers in Chicago and Boston.

Carol S. Weisman, PhD, is Professor of Health Evaluation Sciences and Obstetrics and Gynecology at The Pennsylvania State University College of Medicine, and Director of the Central Pennsylvania Center of Excellence for Research on Pregnancy Outcomes. Dr. Weisman is a sociologist and health services researcher with a principal interest in women's health care and policy. Her research focuses on improving access and quality in women's primary care and on how health risks affect women's health in diverse populations. Dr. Weisman is Editor of the journal *Women's Health Issues*, the peer-reviewed journal of the Jacobs Institute of Women's Health, and she serves on the Institute's Board of Governors. She is the author of over 100 publications, including *Women's Health Care: Activist Traditions and Institutional Change* (Johns Hopkins University Press, 1998).

Dr. Weisman received her Bachelor of Arts from Wellesley College with a major in Sociology and Anthropology, and her Doctorate in Social Relations (Sociology) from The Johns Hopkins University.

Sharon Wallace Williams, PhD, is a research scientist with the Center on Aging and Diversity at the University of North Carolina at Chapel Hill. Dr. Williams received a Bachelor of Science and Master of Science in Communication Disorders, and a Doctorate in Human Development and Family Studies. After her doctoral work, she completed a gerontology postdoctoral fellowship at The Wake Forest University School of Medicine. Her research focuses broadly on chronic disease and the family, with issues of caregiving, social support, and disability at the forefront. Dr. Williams has been involved in research on caregiving and older minority adults, particularly older African Americans. Dr. Williams' current research funding extends her research to include end of life experiences of older adults and family caregivers. Her work has appeared in *The Journal of Gerontology, The Gerontologist, Aging and Mental Health,* and *Family Relations.*

Preface

The health of rural women is of growing concern across the United States, as well as in many other regions of the world. This is because rural women are particularly vulnerable to many health risks. The book addresses the social, economic, and cultural factors that contribute to this elevated risk profile and describes various model programs and best practices designed to lower the health risks associated with being a rural woman in the United States. On top of increased health risks, however, rural women also have to cope with serious limitations in the care that is accessible to them. Many rural areas do not have the specialized health care that is essential for the treatment of serious illnesses, and even basic, primary care is often inadequate. Even when the desired level of health care is available in rural areas, poverty, lack of transportation, and stigmatization often prevent women from receiving the care they need and deserve. A number of possible remedies for dealing with these complicated access issues are described, including policy initiatives and the use of technology.

A unique aspect of the book is its simultaneous focus on the mental, behavioral, and physical health of rural women. Although the prevailing segregation of these areas has been widely recognized as counterproductive, efforts to integrate mental, behavioral, and physical health care have been rewarded with only sporadic success. The causes for this unfortunate state of affairs are complex and include complicated funding and reimbursement practices, professional rivalries and turf battles, and the complexities of linking and integrating different areas of expertise in the interest of providing better health care. Clearly, all health care professionals who serve rural women have a stake in addressing these issues. It is quite fitting, therefore, that the authors of the various chapters of the book include a wide range of health care professionals, including specialists in biobehavioral health, biostatistics, health care economics and health policy research, nursing, nutrition, and pharmacology. In addition, various medical and psychological specialties are represented, as is the field of social work.

All health professional concerned with the health of rural women will benefit from the collective experience and expertise represented in this book. It will also be of particular value in the training of psychologists, social workers, nurses, and physicians who practice or who plan to practice in rural areas. It may also serve as a book of readings in graduate-level courses designed to sensitize aspiring rural health care providers and researchers to the special challenges faced by rural women and to inform them of efforts that are underway across the nation to begin to successfully deal with them. Additionally, it can be used as a set of basic readings on current thinking in the area of rural women's health in continuing education settings. Becoming acquainted with current thinking in the area of rural women's health will help them to become part of future solutions and avoid becoming part of the problem.

The impetus for the development of the book came from the Pennsylvania State University's Rural Women's Health Initiative (RWHI), which is a collaborative undertaking of the Colleges of Agricultural Sciences, Health and Human Development, and Medicine, as well as Outreach and Cooperative Extension. The Initiative was developed to focus national attention on the health concerns of rural women. Since its inception in 1998, the mission of the RWHI has been to improve the quality of health for women of all ages living in rural areas by (1) focusing local, state, and national attention on the health needs of rural women and their families, (2) enhancing the knowledge and skills of the professionals who provide their health care, and (3) disseminating relevant, timely, and useful health information to rural women. Starting in 2000, the Rural Women's Health Initiative developed a number of national conferences to focus attention on generating an interdisciplinary, national dialogue around the mental and physical health concerns of women living in rural America. In 2002, these efforts culminated in a national conference entitled "Linking mental, behavioral, and physical health: Quality of life issues, outcomes, and strategies for health promotion."

Most of the contributions to the present volume resulted from pre-sentations made at this conference, which was held in Washington, D.C. in September of 2002, updated for this volume.

Raymond T. Coward, Ph.D.

Acknowledgments

The present volume owes its existence to the dedication and commitment of the members of Penn State University's Rural Women's Health Initiative. We are grateful for the support of the Penn State community and additional financial support of the conference, which was provided by National Institutes of Health Research Grant #R13-MH66413 from the National Institute of Mental Health and the National Cancer Institute, grant #HHSP233200400433P from the U.S. Department of Health and Human Services Office on Women's Health and Office of Rural Health Policy, and by Eli Lilly and Company. We wish to express our special gratitude to Susan LeWay, Erik Porfeli, and Kim Smith (all of the College of Health and Human Development at Penn State) for supporting the preparation of the manuscript.

Raymond T. Coward, Ph.D.

Introduction

Fred W. Vondracek, Raymond T. Coward, Lisa A. Davis,
Carol H. Gold, Helen Smiciklas-Wright, and
Luanne E. Thorndyke

Health care professionals and researchers have found it convenient and practical to speak of mental, behavioral, and physical health as if they were relatively discreet and separable entities. As more sophisticated conceptual models and analytical tools have become available, however, practitioners and researchers, as well as policy makers, have increased their efforts to link and integrate different levels of analysis and to unify previously segregated areas. Current conceptualizations of human functioning recognize, however, that individuals operate as complex, integrated living systems or "functional units," whose biological structure and physical characteristics make varied behavioral capabilities possible (Ford, 1987). This recognition of the functional relationship between the biological and physical characteristics of the person on the one hand, and the behavior of the person on the other, is central to understanding mental, behavioral, and physical health.

Because "human behavior both shapes and is shaped by the environment" (Ford, 1987), behavior cannot be understood apart from the context within which it occurs. Ultimately, this is the reason that the unique contextual features and social fabric of small towns and rural areas in America contribute significantly to the way people live their lives there, distinct from the patterns found in urban or metropolitan regions. Furthermore, the special contextual features and social fabric of women in rural America is central to understanding the health implications of their mental, behavioral, and physical health. The present volume represents an effort toward interpreting the mental, behavioral, and physical functioning of rural women within their rural environmental context.

BACKGROUND

On September 10, 2001, Tommy Thompson, then Secretary of the U.S. Department of Health and Human Services, released a report from the National Center for Health Statistics that indicated that Americans who live in rural areas rate significantly worse in many key health measures than those who live in the suburbs and in large metropolitan areas. Based on data from the 1990 U.S. Census, 24.8 percent of the population of the United States resided in areas designated as rural, while according to the U.S. Office of Management and Budget (OMB) 20.5 percent of the nation's citizens lived in areas classified as nonmetropolitan (Rural Information Service, 1999). The states with the most rural areas are located in the southern part of the United States, although Pennsylvania, with 3.7 million residents living in areas designated as rural, had the largest rural population of any state in the nation (U.S. Bureau of the Census, 1997).

Although researchers and policy makers continue to encounter some difficulties due to the lack of consistency in the definitions of what constitutes "rural," there is wide agreement that rural populations, regardless of how they are defined, have distinctive characteristics (Coward, Miller, & Dwyer, 1990). Moreover, these distinctive characteristics of rural individuals tend to create differences in their susceptibility to various health problems and in their overall health status. In other words, where one lives can significantly affect one's health because individual health is invariably closely related to the communities and environments in which people live. In fact, one of the underlying assumptions of *Healthy People 2010* is that "the health of the individual is almost inseparable from the health of the larger community" (U.S. Department of Health and Human Services, 1999). Consequently, it is fitting that *Healthy People 2010* has been complemented by *Rural Healthy People 2010*, which calls special attention to the status of health promotion and disease prevention in rural America (Gamm, Hutchison, Dabney, & Dorsey, 2003).

Although individual differences and geographic location have a significant impact on the health of individuals and families, these differences are sometimes overshadowed by biological differences, in particular the sex of the individual. It is well known, for example, that women are twice as likely as men to suffer from major depression, making them more vulnerable to other threats to their health (Barrett, Barrett, Oxman, & Gerber, 1988). They are also more likely than men to suffer from Alzheimer's disease (U.S. Department of Health and Human Services, 1999). Some differences in the health status of women are clearly due to complex interactions among biological, social, and behavioral factors. For example, a number of studies have reported accelerated developmental timetables for rural adolescents, resulting in the early adoption of adult behaviors. For females, this has often meant pregnancy and childbearing during the adolescent years, accompanied by the attendant, usually negative, consequences for educational attainment, social status, and health (Ianni, 1989; Jessor, 1984).

How Are Rural Women Different?

Rural women have distinctive economic characteristics that affect health and well-being. They generally have less formal education than urban women (Bescher-Donnelly & Smith, 1981; Hoppe, 1992; Walker, Walker, & Walker, 1994), and earn about 50 percent less than rural men, while urban women earn only 34 percent less than urban men (Bushy, 1993). Jobs in rural communities tend to be physically demanding, exacerbating generally poor employment prospects for women (Mulder et al., 1999). While poverty rates in rural areas are higher than those in metropolitan areas in all parts of the United States, rural families headed by women (46 percent of rural households) are more likely to be poor than any other type of family (Rogers, 1997). Moreover, because of unemployment, part-time employment necessitated by childcare responsibilities, employment by small private firms, seasonal employment, and many other employment-related factors, rural women are less likely than their urban peers to have health insurance (Bolin & Gamm, 2003). Not surprisingly, poverty and lack of health insurance are associated with a prevalence of chronic conditions, which are then exacerbated by the resulting inadequate access to health care (Broyles, McAuley, & Baird-Holmes, 1999).

Although economic factors are important in determining the health status of rural women, social factors play an equally important role. Rural women marry earlier, bear more children, live in larger families, and hold more conservative family values (Bescher-Donnelly & Smith, 1981; Hoppe, 1992; Brown, 1981; Bushy, 1993; Walker, Walker, & Walker, 1994). They generally outlive their husbands by about 20 years (Bushy, 1993). Nevertheless, in the last decade, rural women entered the work force outside the home to supplement family income and have increased their participation in farm-related work activities. As a result, there has been a corresponding increase in the number of automobile accidents and farm-related injuries involving women. In fact, farm women and children suffer twice as many injuries as do other family members and 70 percent of these injuries are reported as being severe, permanent, or fatal (Bushy, 1993).

According to Bushy (1993), rural women have psychosocial issues that differ from those of their urban counterparts. Despite the multiple connections of family and community, rural women often seem invisible, viewed as an adjunct to their husbands, children, and other family connections. Rural women are more likely to feel that they have a small social network, one that has been disrupted by needing to seek work outside the home or assume more farm-related responsibilities. They are often hesitant to seek support through formal networks because the nature of many small towns and rural communities negates anonymity.

Rural women with children differ significantly from urban women in marital status, level of income, and satisfaction with current life situation. In a study of new mothers in Michigan and Indiana, Walker and colleagues (1994) reported that only 29 percent of rural women had attended college, compared with 53 percent in urban areas, and that they had a lower annual income. Only sixty-five percent of rural women reported being "mostly" or "definitely" satisfied with their current life situation, while 80 percent of urban women reported satisfaction.

Due to biological differences and stressors specific to rural life, rural women face multiple challenges in realizing psychological wellness. In terms of health promotion characteristics, rural women reported less self-actualization and interpersonal support, as well as less healthy nutritional intake. Researchers have also found that socioeconomic factors appeared to increase the risk of poor health outcomes for women living in rural areas (Walker, Walker, & Walker, 1994). The role of rural women presents additional difficulties. Caring for relatives who live in proximity to each other is common for rural women (Bushy, 1993). The results of previous studies have demonstrated psychiatric morbidity to be significantly higher for caregivers within their homes (Horsley, Barrow, Gent, & Astbury, 1998). For those in farming communities, the unpredictability of income brings additional stress (Bushy, 1993). Recent studies have also shown that rural women are more likely to be victims of domestic violence (Krishnan, Hillbert, & Pase, 2001).

Rural Women's Health Status

Rural women utilize prenatal care at lower rates than urban women and birth outcomes are lower in rural areas. Clarke, Farmer, and Miller (1994) reported that in 1988, fewer than 2 percent of all pregnant women in the United States received no prenatal care or entered prenatal care only in the third trimester. In nonmetropolitan areas, however, 16.8 percent of women received inadequate prenatal care, compared with 12.5 percent of women in urban areas. Data from the National Maternal and Infant Health Survey indicated that rural Hispanic women were the least likely to receive prenatal care (Miller, Clarke, Albrecht, & Farmer, 1996). Miller and colleagues postulated that factors contributing to these statistics include poverty, lack of public transportation, and a lack of available health and social services. In a study reported in 1997, researchers compared rural/ urban differences in prenatal care and birth outcomes in a population of women on the mid-Atlantic coast (Alexy, Nichols, Heverly, & Garzon, 1997). The rural group was more likely to be single, less educated, under the age of 18, African American, and have lower annual incomes than the urban cohort. Rural women were more likely to have a poor diet and low pregnancy weight/inadequate weight gain, and to deliver more low birth weight babies.

Persons living in rural areas also experience higher rates of chronic illness and higher death rates due to cardiovascular disease (CVD) than do urban residents (Wright, Champagne, Dever, & Clark,

1985; Edwards, Parker, Burks, West, & Adams, 1991). The largely rural states such as South Carolina, Mississippi, West Virginia, Louisiana, and Georgia have the highest rates of mortality due to CVD (American Heart Association, 1991; Wright, Champagne, Dever, & Clark, 1985). A study published in 1991 investigated rural/urban differences in the prevalence of the four major risk factors for CVD in both African American and White women: elevated blood pressure levels; elevated serum cholesterol levels; smoking; and diabetes. Smoking and diabetes were found to be more common in women living in rural areas; serum cholesterol levels for rural African American women were 11 points above the recommended level. Rates of smoking were 25 to 42 percent higher in rural women than in their urban counterparts (Edwards, Parker, Burks, West & Adams, 1991).

Women in rural areas have been found to be less likely to have had a mammogram than urban women (37 percent compared with 68 percent for women over the age of 50), and only 38 percent of rural women reported ever having a physician recommend mammography as opposed to 65 percent of urban women (Bryant & Mah, 1992; Carr et al., 1996). Researchers conducting focus groups with women living in rural areas reported barriers to breast cancer screening to be cost, transportation, access to facilities, lack of perceived risk, fear, lack of information, and lack of referrals for screening.

Special populations are at particular risk in rural areas of the nation. The rural elderly have poorer health, suffer from more chronic diseases, and are at higher risk for developing nutritional problems than their urban counterparts (Krout, 1986; AbuSabha et al., 1997). Results of a study of the nutritional intake of rural elderly women aged 60–88 years of age who reside in central and eastern Pennsylvania indicated that although 39 percent of the participants rated their health as "good," 60 percent had arthritis, more than two-thirds had high blood pressure, and more than 20 percent indicated heart problems and problems with digestion and circulation. Fifteen percent were diagnosed with diabetes and 14 percent indicated feelings of depression (AbuSabha et al., 1997).

Rural homelessness is a topic not often addressed in the literature. In Wagner, Menke, and Ciccone (1994), researchers noted that homelessness in rural America is largely undocumented, although estimates by the U.S. Department of Housing and Urban Development indicate that the rates of homelessness in rural areas is 6.5/10,000 and the Housing Assistance Council estimated that up to 20 percent of the nation's homeless live in rural areas (Gladden, 1991; Fitchen, 1991). Wagner and her colleagues surveyed 304 homeless women with young children in Ohio to determine their perceived health status and use of health care services. Fifty-three percent of the women had been homeless for 4 to 12 months with 52 percent citing eviction or being left by a partner as the reason for leaving their home. While 83 percent of the women considered themselves to be free of major physical and mental health problems, the most common self-reported health concerns were gynecological disorders (41 percent), headaches (22 percent), allergies (16 percent), and bronchitis (16 percent). Although 62 percent of the women reported having seen a physician within the previous year, 53 percent had not visited a dentist within the previous 12 months. Health risks in the form of drug and alcohol use were indicated for the women participating in the study. Twenty-two percent reported taking prescription drugs, 37 percent used illegal drugs, and almost half reported using alcohol, with 12 percent indicating that they had at least one drink per day. Seventy-four percent smoked cigarettes.

Barriers to Adequate Health Care for Rural Women

Rural women, by and large, do not receive adequate health care. Although most experts agree on this, the reasons for this deficiency are complex and multifaceted. Barriers to adequate health care for rural women include obstacles that are external in nature, such as policies related to insurability and eligibility, and internal, such as belief systems, fears, and anxieties.

Even though over 20 percent of the U.S. population lives in rural areas, less than 10 percent of the nation's physicians practice in rural America. Particularly telling is the fact that the rural supply of physicians lags far behind the urban supply, and that virtually all specialty-trained physicians are much more likely to practice in urban areas and rural areas adjacent to urban areas (Rosenblatt & Hart, 1999). For rural women, this is particularly critical with regard to availability of obstetricians/gynecologists. In rural counties without even moderate-sized cities, there are currently fewer than three obstetricians/gynecologists per 100,000 residents (Rosenblatt & Hart, 1999).

While mental and behavioral health services are necessary throughout the nation, they are often even more difficult to obtain than general medical services or are altogether unavailable for residents of rural areas. Mental health providers are in short supply, and primary care physicians may not provide these services (Bird, Lambert, & Hartley, 1995). Obstacles to receiving mental health services also include poor roads and distance barriers (U.S. Department of Health and Human Services, 1999; Beeson, Britain, Howell, Kirwan, & Sawyer, 1998). A recent study has shown that individuals in rural populations do not seek out services, even when educational interventions are extended to help raise awareness of symptoms (Fox, Blank, Rovnyak, & Barnett, 2001).

Although rural areas are considered to be tranquil and carefree, rural residents experience mental health problems as frequently as urban residents (Philbrick, Connelly, & Wofford, 1996). Alcohol and drug abuse are, in most cases, as high in rural areas as in urban areas, and in some cases even higher (Hartley, Bird, & Dempsey, 1999). All of the major diseases, from heart disease and stroke to diabetes and cancer, are identified by people living in rural areas as significant health concerns (Gamm, Hutchison Dabney, & Dorsey, 2003). The existing barriers to adequate health care for rural women thus exacerbate the health problems that are experienced. Access is clearly not the only obstacle, however, as belief systems among individuals in rural America must be addressed as well, using understanding and education (Hoyt, Conger, Valde, & Wiehs, 1997).

PLAN OF THE BOOK

In 1997, to focus scientific attention on the health of rural women, several units of The Pennsylvania State University formed what has come to be known as the "Penn State Rural Women's Health Initiative"—including the College of Agricultural Science, Cooperative Extension, the College of Health and Human Development, and the College of Medicine. As observed by the president of the University (Spanier, 2001), the benefit of such a partnership is that it can transcend disciplinary boundaries to address the problems faced by society, "cross state and regional lines to share information, give critical mass and momentum to advocacy, and promote research, education, and service delivery." As part of its mission to share information about rural women's health, the initiative organized a number of national conferences. The first conference took place in Washington, D.C. in 2000. It was followed in 2002 by a second conference, also in Washington, with the theme "Rural Women's Health: Linking Mental, Behavioral, and Physical Health." Most of the chapters prepared for the present volume are an outgrowth of that conference.

The first five chapters are designed to introduce the reader to the breadth and depth of issues facing rural women compared with their peers in urban and metropolitan environments. In chapter 1, Mulder and Lambert provide an overview of the stressors and challenges that have a unique impact on the health and well-being of rural women. Chapter 2 is devoted to a provocative review of policy issues that specifically address the circumstances of rural women. In that chapter, McNamara presents a framework for considering policy changes that have the potential for making a positive difference in the lives of rural women in the next decade. In Chapter 3, Gold and colleagues highlight a problem that has been particularly difficult to address in rural populations in general, and among older rural women in particular, namely the problem of availability and utilization of mental health treatment. Olson and Bove highlight another significant health problem for rural women in Chapter 4 by focusing on obesity and the multiple risk factors associated with this increasingly pervasive health problem. In Chapter 5, Hillemeier, Weisman, Chase, and Darnell examine the problems of preterm birth and low birth weight among rural women, discuss risk factors that are of particular concern among rural women, and conclude by describing an innovative approach to the prevention of preterm birth and low birth weight (and the attendant health consequences) in this population.

Chapters 6 through 8 examine barriers to the care and treatment of rural women in the critically important area of mental health. In Chapter 6, Bolin demonstrates that rural women with chronic mental health challenges have reduced work and lower wages when compared with their urban peers. Bolin observes not only that rural women are worse off than their urban counterparts, but that rural women in the south and west fare worse than their counterparts in other parts of the country and that minority rural women in these areas are even more disadvantaged regarding opportunities for working, wages, and access to health insurance. In Chapter 7, Shinogle uses data from the Medical Expenditure Panel Survey to examine patterns of rural women's utilization and expenditures for mental health and substance abuse treatment, finding that rural women, and particularly African-American rural women, are less likely to use substance abuse and mental health services than their urban counterparts, even when controlling for demographic factors and self-reported mental health status. In another study that uses a different set of empirical data regarding the utilization of mental health services by rural women, Gehlert and her collaborators observe in chapter 8 that negative attitudes toward mental health services (including fear of stigmatization) may be the most important impediment to actually seeking and obtaining such services.

Chapters 9, 10, and 11 examine special populations among rural women at risk for poor health outcomes. In chapter 9, Campbell, Bursac, and Perkins report on risk factors for the health of rural American Indian women in Oklahoma. Among other things, they observe that smoking, being overweight, and physical inactivity are the primary risk factors that should be addressed in health promotion and disease prevention programs with this population. Goodwin and colleagues examined very specific populations, namely African American rural and urban women who are caregivers to dependent elderly. Presenting their findings in chapter 10, they note that informal personal, social, and economic resources are important to both urban and rural women who are exposed to particularly heavy role demands because of their care giving activities. In chapter 11, Probst and colleagues examine the effects of race and poverty on perceived stress in rural women. They found that rural women did not report greater levels of stress than urban women, leading them to suggest that a fruitful avenue for future research might be to explore unique sources of support and resilience in rural areas.

In Chapters 12 and 13, two authors offer a selective look at prevention and intervention methodologies that promise to be effective in improving the health status of rural women. In chapter 12, Parrett describes a combined nutrition education and exercise intervention for rural elders (mostly women) who live in a government subsidized apartment complex. Although her findings are limited by the small sample size and the relative brevity of the intervention, they point to a model of intervention that has promise for improving both the mental and physical functioning (and thus the general health) of elderly women. Moving from the level of intervening with individuals or small groups, Jameson addresses the systemic problem of providing quality health care to a geographically dispersed rural population in Chapter 13. Using the Inland Northwest Health Services in predominantly rural Eastern Washington as an example, she documents how collaboration instead of competition, as well as the use of technology, increases the reach, efficiency, and effectiveness of health care providers in rural regions of the country.

In the final chapter, Thorndyke provides an integrative summary of the diverse findings on rural women's health that are presented throughout this volume. Although the summary demonstrates the advantages of the joint consideration of rural women's mental, behavioral, and physical health, it also highlights the urgent need for increased research efforts in this important area. Specifically, Thorndyke recommends a sharper focus on well defined, specific rural populations, an increased emphasis on outcomes-based research and on identifying factors that contribute to the resiliency of rural women, and the development of a better understanding of factors necessary to attract, support, and retain health care service providers in rural areas. It is the editors' hope that the present volume will serve to inspire others to join ongoing efforts to address these issues in the interest of advancing the health of rural women throughout the nation.

REFERENCES

AbuSabha, R., Wright, H. S., Jensen, G. L., Achterberg, C., Harkness, W., & vonEye, A. (1997). Factors associated with diet and weight in rural older women. *Journal of Nutrition for the Elderly, 16*(3), 1–16.

Alexy, B., Nichols, B., Heverly, M. A., & Garzon, L. (1997). Prenatal factors and birth outcomes in the public health service: A rural/urban comparison. *Research in Nursing & Health, 20*(1), 61–70.

American Heart Association (1991). *Heart facts.* Dallas: American Heart Association Office of Communications.

Barrett, J. E., Barrett, J. A., Oxman, T. E., & Gerber, P. D. (1988). The prevalence of psychiatric disorders in a primary care practice. *Archives of General Psychiatry, 45*, 1100–1106.

Beeson, P. G., Britain, C., Howell, M. L., Kirwan, D., & Sawyer, D. A. (1998). Rural mental health at the millennium. In R. W. Mandersheid & M. J. Henderson (Eds.), *Mental Health United States, 1998* (DHHS Publication No. SMA 99-3285). Washington, DC: U.S. Government Printing Office.

Bescher-Donnelly, L., & Smith, L. W. (1981). The changing roles and status of rural women. In R. T. Coward & W. M. Smith (Eds.), *The family in rural society.* Boulder, CO: Westview Press.

Bird, D. C., Lambert, D., & Hartley, D. (1995). Rural models for integrating primary care, mental health, and substance abuse treatment services. Retrieved October 13, 2004 from http://muskie.usm.maine.edu/ihp/ruralheal/index.jsp

Bolin, J., & Gamm, L. D. (2003). Access to quality health services in rural areas— insurance: A literature review. In L. D. Gamm, L. L. Hutchison, B. J. Dabney, & A. M. Dorsey (Eds.), *Rural healthy people 2010: A companion document to healthy people 2010, 2,* 5–16. College Station, TX: The Texas A&M University System Health Sciences Center, School of Rural Public Health, Southwest Rural Health Research Center.

Brown, D. L. (1981). A quarter century of trends and changes in the demographic structure of American Families. In R. T. Coward & W. M. Smith (Eds.), *The family in rural society.* Boulder, CO: Westview Press.

Broyles, R. W., McAuley, W. J., & Baird-Holmes, D. (1999). The medically vulnerable: Their health risks, health status, and use of physician care. *Journal of Health Care for the Poor and Underserved, 10*(2), 186–200.

Bryant, H., & Mah, Z. (1992). Breast cancer screening attitudes and behaviors of rural and urban women. *Preventive Medicine, 21*(4), 405–418.

Bushy, A. (1993). Rural women: Lifestyle and health status. *Nursing Clinics of North America, 28*(1), 187–197.

Carr, W. P., Maldonado, G., Leonard, P. R., Halberg, J. U., Church, T. R., Mandel, J. H., et al. (1996). Mammogram utilization among farm women. *The Journal of Rural Health, 22*(4), 278–290.

Clarke, L. L., Farmer, F. I., & Miller, M. K. (1994). Structural determinants of infant mortality in metropolitan and nonmetropolitan America. *Rural Sociology, 59*(1), 84–99.

Coward, R. T., Miller, M. K., & Dwyer, J. W. (1990). Rural America in the 1980s: A context for rural health research. *The Journal of Rural Health, 6*(4), 357–363.

Edwards, K. A., Parker, D. E., Burks, C. D., West, A. M., & Adams, M. (1991). Cardiovascular risks: Among black and white rural-urban low-income women. *The Association of Black Nursing Faculty Journal, 2*(4), 72–76.

Fitchen, J. M. (1991). Homelessness and landlessness: Perspectives from Upstate New York. *Urban Anthropology, 20*(2), 177–210.

Ford, D. H. (1987). *Humans as self-constructing living systems: A developmental perspective on behavior and personality.* Hillsdale, NJ: Lawrence Erlbaum Associates.

Fox, J. C., Blank, M. B., Rovnyak, V. G., & Barnett, R. Y. (2001). Barriers to help seeking for mental disorders in a rural impoverished population. *Community Mental Health Journal, 37*(5), 421–436.

Gamm, L. D., Hutchison, L. L., Dabney, B. J., & Dorsey, A. M. (2003). *Rural healthy people 2010: A companion document to healthy people 2010, 2.* College Station,

TX: The Texas A&M University System Health Sciences Center, School of Rural Public Health, Southwest Rural Health Research Center.

Gladden, J. (1991). Homelessness: A rural perspective. In A. Busby (Ed.), *Rural Nursing, Vol. 1.* Newbury Park, CA: Sage Publications.

Hartley, D., Bird, D. C., & Dempsey, P. (1999). Rural mental health and substance abuse. In T. C. Ricketts, III (Ed.), *Rural health in the United States.* New York: Oxford University Press.

Hoppe, R. (1992). Household income remains lower in rural areas. *Rural Conditions and Trends, 3*(1), 14–15.

Horsley, S., Barrow, S., Gent, N., & Astbury, J. (1998). Informal care and psychiatric morbidity. *Journal of Public Health Medicine, 20*(2), 180–185.

Hoyt, D. R., Conger, R. D., Valde, J. G., & Wiehs, K. (1997). Psychological distress and help seeking in rural America. *American Journal of Community Psychology, 25*(4), 449–470.

Ianni, F. A. J. (1989). *The search for structure: A report on American youth today.* New York: Free Press.

Jessor, R. (1984). Adolescent development and behavioral health. In J. D. Matarazzo, S. M. Weiss, J. A. Herd, N. E. Miller, & S. M. Weiss (Eds.), *Behavioral health: A handbook of health enhancement and disease prevention.* New York: Wiley.

Krishnan, S. P., Hillbert, J. C., & Pase, M. (2001). An examination in intimate partner violence in rural communities: Results from a hospital emergency department study from southwest United States. *Family and Community Health, 24*(1), 1–14.

Krout, J. A. (1986). *The aged in rural America.* Westport, CT: Greenwood Press.

Miller, M. K., Clarke, L. L., Albrecht, S. L., & Farmer, F. L. (1996). The interactive effects of race and ethnicity and mother's residence on the adequacy of prenatal care. *The Journal of Rural Health, 12*(1), 6–18.

Mulder, P. L., Kenkel, M. B., Shellenberger, S., Constantine, M. G., Streiegel, R., Sears, S. F., Jr., et al. (1999). *Behavioral health care needs of rural women: Report of the Rural Women's Work Group.* Available from the American Psychological Association web site at http://www.apa.org/rural/ruralwomen.pdf

Philbrick, J. T., Connelly, J. E., & Wofford, A. B. (1996). The prevalence of mental disorders in rural office practice. *Journal of General Internal Medicine, 1*(1), 9–15.

Rogers, C. C. (1997). Nonmetro elders better off than metro elders on some measures but not on others. *Rural Conditions and Trends, 8*(2), 52–59.

Rosenblatt, R. A., & Hart, L. G. (1999). Physicians and rural America. In T. C. Ricketts, III (Ed.), *Rural health in the United States.* New York: Oxford University Press.

Rural Information Service (1999). Facts About the Rural Population of the United States. Retrieved October 4, 2004 from http://www.nal.usda.gov/ric/richs/stats/htlm

Spanier, G. B. (2001). Bridging rural women's health into the new millennium. *Women's Health Issues, 11*(1), 2–6.

U.S. Bureau of the Census (1997). *Table 3: Distribution of the Population, by Region, Residence, Sex, and Race: March 1996.* Retrieved June 26, 2004 from http://www.census.gov/population/socdemo/race/black/tabs96/tab03-96.txt

U.S. Department of Health and Human Services (1999). *Mental Health: A Report of the Surgeon General—Executive Summary.* Rockville, MD: U.S. Department of Health and Human Services.

Wagner, J. D., Menke, E. M., & Ciccone, J. K. (1994). The health of rural homeless women with young children. *The Journal of Rural Health, 10*(1), 49–57.

Walker, L. O, Walker, M. L., & Walker, M. E. (1994). Health and well-being of childbearing women in rural and urban contexts. *The Journal of Rural Health, 10*(3), 168–172.

Wright, J. S., Champagne, F., Dever, G. E., & Clark, F. C. (1985). A comparative analysis of rural and urban mortality. *American Journal of Preventive Medicine, 1,* 22–29.

Chapter 1

Behavioral Health of Rural Women: Challenges and Stressors

Pamela L. Mulder and Warren Lambert

Thirty percent of American women or about one woman in three, lives in a region or area defined as rural (Bergland, 1988). These women are not a single homogeneous group; they can be found in every state and among them are representatives of virtually every ethnic, cultural, and socioeconomic group. Their personal situations are varied and individual. Nonetheless, these diverse women often experience many similar environmental, social, and economic challenges as a consequence of their rural residency. These common challenges are the stressors that have an impact on the mental and physical health of rural women and that uniquely influence the epidemiology, presentation, and treatment of the disorders that arise.

Rural women experience mental and physical illness at rates that equal, and in some cases exceed, those of urban residents, but rural women frequently lack access to both health care options and various supportive, ancillary services available in more metropolitan settings. Moreover, although rural women comprise a sizable population across the United States, they lack political power, and their needs and concerns are frequently overlooked by policy makers.

This chapter provides an overview of many of the stressors and challenges commonly experienced by many rural women. Because this topic is quite broad, the stressors and challenges have been organized into three groups, artificially distinguishing among those that are largely socioeconomic in nature, those that are primarily sociocultural, and those that are specifically health concerns (including physical, emotional, and behavioral health issues). These stressors are discussed in terms of discrepancies between urban and rural etiology and the unique impact of rural residence on incidence or presentation.

These stressors and challenges are interrelated aspects of a rural environment. It is not reasonable to assume that the stressors are always "causes" rather than "effects." For example, although behavioral health problems are often presented as if they were "outcomes," it is clear that poor health is, in fact, a stressor. Moreover, even if a particular stressor or challenge is clearly causal in a given situation, it is very difficult to predict the precise behavioral outcomes across situations. Humans are complex, "self constructing" organisms, and very similar events and experiences may produce any of a number of outcomes (the principle of equipotentiality) depending on the strengths and vulnerabilities of given individuals and their situations (Ford & Lerner, 1992).

A hypothetical, but representative, case history will be used to illustrate the interrelated nature and potential impact of these stressors on rural women's emotional and behavioral health. The case of Sharon Adkins (not her real name) and her family, described below, illustrates many of the socioeconomic, sociocultural, and behavioral health challenges often encountered by rural women. This case also illustrates the interrelated nature of these factors as Sharon's story is continued in each of the relevant sections of this chapter.

> The Adkins household consists of five persons, including Sharon (age 48), her husband Tom (age 56), their daughter Tammy (age 19), Tammy's daughter Mary (age 18 months), and Sharon's mother, Anne (age 68). The family lives in a 3-bedroom mobile home in an isolated, mountainous hollow served by one tertiary [gravel] road. The nearest neighbor lives three miles farther up

the hill and the nearest town is at the base of the hill, 8 miles down the road. There is one small combination convenience store pharmacy post office in the town. The community mental health center, regional hospital, and social services offices are all at least 40 miles away in another county. Sharon presents with symptoms of depression and anxiety. She is concerned about the family's poor finances, her husband's abuse of alcohol, the poor educational and career options available to her children, her mother's failing health, and, lastly, her own well-being.

COMMON STRESSORS AND CHALLENGES OF RURAL LIFE

Socioeconomic challenges faced by many rural residents include high rates of poverty, unemployment, and limited educational and vocational opportunities. Sociocultural stressors and challenges that rural women frequently encounter include role overload, isolation, patriarchal social structures, a lack of anonymity, and the lack of social support services. Behavioral health issues that are common problems in rural areas include high rates of tobacco, alcohol, and other substance abuse, obesity, a sedentary lifestyle, lack of preventive self-care, depression and anxiety, family and interpersonal violence, accidents, lack of access to primary and specialized health care, and a lack of medical insurance coverage.

Socioeconomic Stressors

Sharon is a high-school graduate, but she has never been employed outside the home. Tom has been unemployed since he sustained a back injury on a logging job about 3 years ago. Sharon's older daughter, Tammy, became pregnant at the age of 16 and quit school to marry the father. After suffering physical abuse, Tammy moved back into her parents' home with her daughter. Tammy is not employed, has no income, and cannot afford the cost of filing for divorce. The family's monthly income consists of Tom's monthly disability payment ($623) and Anne's social security payment ($321).

Unemployment in the area is very high; local jobs that pay decently and offer any benefits are almost all labor-intensive mining and logging work. There is little opportunity for women to work outside the home. There are no daycare centers where working women can enroll their young children. Some of the women in the community do care for children in their homes, but openings are very rare and the relatively few local women who do work outside their homes depend on family members to provide child care.

Poverty, unemployment, and a scarcity of resources are common problems in many rural communities. The majority of the most seriously and persistently impoverished counties in the United States are rural counties. Ninety-five percent of the persistent poverty counties (poverty rates of greater than 20 percent during all decades from 1960 to 2000) in the United States are nonmetropolitan, and more than 70 percent of these counties are specifically classified as rural (Miller, 2003).

The rural poverty rate varies with family structure, marital status, and ethnicity. Recent surveys by the United States Department of Agriculture (USDA) show that more than half (56.9 percent) of all rural families with children younger than 18 years of age have annual incomes below the poverty line. Rural families headed by women experience greater poverty than those headed by males. Thirty-five percent of rural families with a female head of household are classified as living in poverty—nearly four times the rate for families with a male head of household. Nearly one-third (30.4 percent) of rural women living alone are also poor; the nonmetropolitan poverty rate for single females is almost 9 percentage points higher than the rate for single metropolitan females (U.S. Department of Agriculture, 2000). In terms of ethnicity, although two-thirds of the rural poor are non-Hispanic Caucasians (the greatest proportion of this diverse population), poverty levels are highest for ethnic minority women, particularly for those living in the rural southeastern United States (USDA, 1998).

Twenty-six percent of American women with disabilities live in rural communities and they tend to be poorer (80 percent make less than $10,000 a year), less-educated, and more dependent on government social service programs than other rural residents (Seekins, Innes, & Maxon, 1998). Rural women with disabilities are approximately three times less likely to be employed (27 percent) than rural women without disabilities. In comparison, rural men with disabilities are approximately two times less likely to be employed (38 percent) than men without disabilities (Seekins, Innes, & Maxon, 1998).

Elderly women, who are disproportionately represented in rural communities, experience the most severe poverty (Seekins, Innes, & Maxon, 1998). Nonmetropolitan elders have significantly higher rates of poverty than their metropolitan counterparts; they represent 20.3 percent of those in poverty, compared with 13.5 percent in metro areas (Centers for Disease Control, 1997). The average income was $8,209 per year for elderly rural women versus an urban average of $11,869 (Schwenk, 1994). Poverty rates are even higher for disabled elderly rural women (Seekins, Innes, & Maxon, 1998). As is the case with rural women in general, the economic status of rural elderly is correlated with marital status. Eight percent of elderly rural couples were poor, but more than 33 percent of single or widowed women have annual incomes below the poverty level (Glasgow, Holden, McLaughlin, & Rowles, 1993).

Rural women have few resources to call upon to relieve their poverty. On average, rural women have fewer years of education and earn lower wages than their urban counterparts (Bhatta, 2001). Rural economies are often based on male-dominated, labor-intensive industries such as mining, agriculture, logging, and fishing; in recent years, service jobs have begun to develop in many rural regions, but these offer very low wages (Rojewski, Wicklein, & Schell, 1995). Childcare options, public transportation, and job training programs are limited or entirely absent in most rural communities (Beck, Jijon, & Edwards, 1996).

Sociocultural Stressors

Sharon feels responsible for caring for all of her family members and assigns greater priority to their needs and wishes than to her own. Her mother Anne has serious health problems and her condition has worsened rapidly during the past two years. Anne moved into her daughter's home two years ago with the expectation that Sharon would provide the needed care herself, but now requires constant supervision and frequent emergency medical intervention. Sharon complains of not having sufficient strength to "keep doing it all" and when she is asked about support systems and resources, she says that her church and her faith sustain her.

To help make ends meet, Sharon maintains a small vegetable garden, makes her own jellies, and cans many of the vegetables that she grows. She keeps chickens for eggs but recently sold the family's other livestock (two pigs, a nanny goat, and a cow) because her mother's care demanded so much of her time and Tom's unemployment left the family unable to cover the veterinary and food costs.

Anonymity is entirely lacking in this small, close-knit community. Tammy's brother-in-law was the law enforcement officer dispatched to her home the night that she was beaten by her husband. There used to be a "safe house" for abused women in the area. Before it closed, almost anyone could have given a newcomer the address. Sharon's minister frequently exhorts her to try to convince Tom to attend the weekly AA meeting at the church and even indicates several men in the congregation that he is sure Tom knows who would be there to make him feel welcome.

The cultural attitudes in rural communities frequently include a preference for self-reliance, distrust of strangers, stigmatization of persons with certain types of mental or physical illness, acceptance of self-perceived poor health, and a pervading patriarchal (male-dominated) traditionalism that defies social change (Bushy, 1993; Wagenfeld, Murray, Mohatt, & Debruyn, 1993). These attitudes, which thrive in an environment characterized by dense social relationships and strong kinship ties, frequently become barriers to intervention and treatment because they result in a lack of anonymity, potentially compromised confidentiality, and, often, questionable provider objectivity.

One impact of a patriarchal social structure is the division of labor by sex. Specific activities are clearly considered to be "women's work." Rural women are typically the "backbone" of their families and their communities. They are typically married and provide care for large extended families. They tend to have their first children at younger ages than urban women (Frenzen & Butler, 1997). Rural women are likely to be fully responsible for children and the care of the home (usually with little or no assistance from spouses); they are also responsible for the care of sick, elderly, or disabled family members and often for other community residents as well (Bushy, 1993). They are the volunteers upon which communities, churches, and social agencies often rely.

Role overload is one of the common stressors encountered by rural women. In addition to their roles as homemakers, many of these women also have responsibilities related to a family business, farm maintenance, livestock care, or home gardening. The related duties may range from the deskwork of bookkeeping to heavy labor, canning, tilling, planting, harvesting, and paraveterinary tasks. Added to these responsibilities, financial constraints lead many rural women to seek employment outside the home. This form of role overload has been referred to as "the third-shift phenomenon" (Gallagher & Delworth, 1993; Meadows, Thurston, & Berenson, 2001).

Isolation is often imposed on rural residents as a result of geographic barriers or simply the widely distributed homesteads often found in sparsely populated areas. The nearest neighbor may be more than walking distance away. At the same time, anonymity is often lacking in small rural communities where most of the residents know one another well. This isolation, added to the lack of anonymity and the predominance of patriarchal traditions often associated with the rural lifestyle, can have a unique impact on the rural woman's health and well-being. For example, as will be noted in the following section, spousal abuse, suicide, and homicide are serious problems in rural communities. However, factors like isolation, lack of anonymity, patriarchal cultural traditions, added to the lack of support services in many communities, limit the alternatives available to victims of violence (Anahita, 1998). Geographical isolation lessens the probability that the violent behavior will be witnessed by a third party and, because rural communities are often structured around a few large extended families and a complex interweaving of economic and social ties, it is not uncommon for the offender to be related to law enforcement personnel and emergency responders, potentially limiting the victim's ability to obtain objective assistance. Many rural women have refrained from seeking assistance because of the negative impact of gossip and stigma on family members, and it is not uncommon for senior women in a rural family to discourage younger women from reporting abuse by marginalizing or "normalizing" the violence as something that should be expected and endured (Mulder & Chang, 1997). The lack of anonymity in rural communities may also result in under-reporting of suicides because rural coroners may be reticent to specify suicide as the actual cause of a woman's death, preferring to protect the feelings of immediate family members or to avoid religious or ideological implications and social stigma in a small community (Greenberg, Carey, & Popper, 1987). One eventual result of this type of biased reporting is that the actual level of unmet mental and behavioral health need is not accurately documented and interventions are not readily forthcoming.

Stressors Related to Physical, Emotional, and Behavioral Health

> All four of the adults in the house smoke cigarettes. Sharon has become concerned about the effects of second-hand smoke on little Mary, and she and Tammy have restricted themselves to smoking outside. Tom is less cooperative, especially when he has been drinking, and Sharon says that he slapped her the last time she suggested that he consider changing his behavior. Sharon describes their lifestyle as very sedentary, mostly sitting and watching television. Despite Sharon's garden and the eggs laid by the chickens, the family diet consists largely of low-cost, bulky starches (pastas, rice, and potatoes) prepared with reusable lards; all four adults in the family are obese.
>
> Sharon is also concerned because she felt a" lump" in her right breast about four months ago. She saw the family doctor but has not yet been able to schedule a mammogram, which would require traveling across the county to the regional hospital. Because the family does not have an automobile, Sharon has to pay a neighbor to take the family members to town for shopping and appointments with the family doctor. She is very concerned about how she will care for her family if she needs to undergo surgery or any series of chemical or radiation treatments. She describes her concerns about the travel requirements, her duties at home, and the cost of her care as being overwhelming.

Rural women are at very great risk for depression and stress related disorders (Beck, Jijon, & Edwards, 1996; Centers for Disease Control, 1997; Van Hightower & Dorsey, 2001) and although many studies suggest that these disorders may be more common among rural women than urban women, they are less likely to be diagnosed by rural practitioners (Rost, Williams, Wherry, & Smith, 1995). Rural women discuss the symptoms of depression with their primary care providers less frequently, and more often present in primary care settings with psychosomatic symptoms such as headaches, backaches, insomnia, fatigue, and abdominal pain (Van Hook, 1996). Depressive symptoms among rural women are frequently found to be correlated with greater poverty, less education, and being unmarried (Van Hook, 1996).

In comparison to urbanites, rural women of all ages generally suffer from higher incidences of chronic illness and experience greater disability and morbidity related to diabetes, cancer, hypertension, heart disease, stroke, and lung disease (Centers for Disease Control, 1997; Duelberg, 1992; U.S. Department of Agriculture, 1997). Some of the reasons for these high rates may be sociocultural. For example, rural women are more likely to smoke, even during pregnancy, and to be obese; they are also less likely to exercise than women in more urban settings (Duelberg, 1992). They also have higher rates of alcohol abuse and dependence than urban women, and are more likely to report bouts of heavy drinking (Donnermeyer, 1995). Other reasons for the high rates may include a lack of knowledge about early detection and prevention measures, inability to access treatment options, or disbelief concerning the efficacy of various interventions. Both rural and urban women have been found to perceive their preventive care needs as being unjustified additional burdens on overworked primary care physicians (Meadows, Thurston, & Berenson, 2001). Rural women typically undergo PAP smears less often than urban women and are less likely to have had regular mammograms. Therefore, many health problems are in advanced stages by the time rural women seek out medical care, resulting in poorer prognoses and requiring more aggressive treatment (Duelberg, 1992). Factors that are unique to rural residence also limit women's treatment choices. Discharge data from the Hospital Cost and Utilization Project (1981–1987) show that women treated in urban hospitals are nearly twice as likely to have a breast-conserving procedure and 40 percent less likely to have a radical mastectomy than patients who are from rural areas or who are treated in rural facilities (Khojasteh, Westhoff, Hackman, & Stone, 1999). The rural women surveyed in that study cited transportation as a major factor in this decision process, indicating that they anticipate problems traveling on icy rural roads to complete radiation (and other) treatments associated with lumpectomy and similar procedures (Khojasteh, Westhoff, Hackman, & Stone, 1999).

Many other sex-specific sexual and reproductive health problems are also critical concerns for rural women. Fetal, infant, and maternal mortality are all disproportionately high in rural regions (United States Congress Office of Technology Assessment, 1990) and a greater proportion of rural births is to teenage mothers (Frenzen & Butler, 1997). Several studies indicate that, in comparison with urban women, rural women seriously underestimate the risk of HIV infection (National Rural Health Association, 1997) at a time when the highest rate of increased incidence is among African American women living in impoverished rural counties in the southeastern United States (Crosby, Yarber, DiClemente, Wingood, & Meyerson, 2002). Men who live in rural areas were found to be less likely to use condoms than were those living in large metropolitan areas; a large percentage of these men also indicated that they engaged in extramarital heterosexual encounters in urban areas without their wives' knowledge (Anderson, Wilson, Doll, Jones, & Barker, 1999). Given the patriarchal social milieu commonly found in rural communities, rural women may be unlikely to insist on what may seem to be an unnecessary use of condoms. Rural women, single or married, may be reluctant to purchase condoms in local pharmacies, fearing the implications of such a purchase in a social climate where anonymity is often lacking.

Violence against women, including spousal abuse, homicide, and even suicide are all serious problems in rural communities. Rates of spousal/intimate partner abuse and the incidence of completed rape are as high in rural areas as in urban (Donnermeyer, 1995; Rennison & Welchans, 2000). Overall suicide rates are highest in rural areas of the western states, with young women in this region committing suicide three times more often than those living in metropolitan settings (Centers for Disease Control, 1997; Greenberg, Carey, & Popper, 1987). Young rural women who commit suicide are more likely to employ firearms (Greenberg, Carey, & Popper, 1987; National Center for Injury Prevention and Control, 1998). Both homicides and suicides occur disproportionately among young Native Americans living in rural areas and homicide is the third leading cause of death for Native American females 15 to 34 years of age (National Center for Injury Prevention and Control, 1998). Rural residence has been associated with higher rates of homicide throughout the United States (Centers for Disease Control, 1997).

Rural women may also suffer from the hazards of employment specific to rural environments. For example, high rates of non-Hodgkin's lymphoma, leukemia, multiple myeloma, and cancers of the breast, ovary, lung, bladder, and cervix have been reported for female farm workers exposed to agricultural chemicals (McDuffie, 1994). Secondary exposure to these toxins while laundering clothing worn by agriculture workers also poses considerable risk to rural women (Grieshop, Villanueva, & Stiles, 1994).

Rural women are also more likely than urban residents to be involved in an injury-producing accident (Agency for Health Care Policy and Research, 1996). Traumatic injuries are more common in rural areas, and rural residents face worse outcomes and higher risks of death than urban patients, partly because of transportation problems and lack of advanced life-support training for emergency medical personnel (Agency for Health Care Policy and Research, 1996).

Lack of health insurance and the lack of access to health care services are among the most significant stressors cited by rural women. Although rural women commonly describe the geographic and/or temporal barriers that they face in terms of accessing the health care system from a rural residence, the cost of health care is by far the most dominant barrier cited (Meadows, Thurston, & Berenson, 2001). Rural residents, particularly rural women, are less likely to be insured than their urban counterparts and both the women themselves and their health care providers are more dependent on receiving Medicare for services than urban residents (Seccombe, 1995; U.S. Department of Agriculture, 1998). Low-income elders living in rural areas are nearly twice as likely to receive Medicaid and rely on this service as a sole supplement to Medicare than those elderly living in urban areas (Seccombe, 1995).

Access to care and availability of services are problems in rural areas. As of 1996, 60 percent of the rural counties in the U.S. were designated as Medically Underserved Areas (MUAs) because of the lack of access to primary health care. There are very few readily accessible medical specialists outside the area of family medicine in rural areas. In addition, 55 percent of all U.S. counties are not served by a psychiatrist, a psychologist, or a social worker, and all of these unserved counties are rural (National Advisory Committee on Rural Health, 1993).

The lack of services and treatment options, the dearth of both primary and specialty health care professionals, added to difficulties associated with cost, lack of transportation, lack of child care or coverage for many other culturally mandated duties demanded of rural women at home or on farms are formidable barriers to service provision in rural communities where the unmet need is often significant, although not necessarily accurately documented.

FINAL COMMENTS AND RECOMMENDATIONS FOR THE FUTURE

Until recently, rural concerns have not been a priority for federal agencies and policy makers. Rural residence has not been a commonly noted research demographic and, when this variable has been included, it has rarely been further defined in terms of age, sex, and ethnicity. Current research focused on the behavioral health care concerns of specific subgroups of rural women (such as lesbian/ bisexual women, women with disabilities, and women who are migrant farm workers) is likely to add significantly to this growing literature base. Questions about the efficacy of rural implementation of social programs and interventions designed for use in more urban settings are now being considered, including the efficacy of various federal policies that may have an impact on rural behavioral health. Training curricula and internship sites oriented towards rural areas are being developed to prepare health care providers to address the unmet needs of rural residents in culturally sensitive ways.

One of the many research directions offering significant potential benefit to rural women is the topic of resiliency. This chapter has been focused on stressors and challenges that rural women commonly experience with a clear implication that any or all of these factors may have a negative impact on the women's health and well-being. These are legitimate concerns that require attention. However, it is all too easy to overlook the obvious reality that these women have been managing these stressors for generations. These are strong, self-reliant women who truly are the community caregivers and volunteers. Many of the factors that have been presented as stressors, including the cultural milieu of close relationships among extended family members, may also contribute to the rural woman's strength and resiliency. There is growing evidence suggesting that many rural women feel strengthened by their involvement with their community, their attachments to others in the community, and their opportunities to care for one another. Rural women are not only the ideal pool from which to draw indigenous lay health care workers (and future professionals), this involvement may be beneficial to participants themselves in multiple ways, providing outlets for involvement and also a potential for further education and additional income. In terms of the development of effective intervention and prevention models, it will be important for future investigators to focus on identifying factors that may contribute to the rural woman's physical and emotional well-being as opposed to diagnosing and treating illness. It would also be appropriate to consider the rural woman's spiritual wellness as a resiliency variable, given a frequently noted reliance on religious support systems (Mulder & Chang, 1977).

Sparsely populated and often impoverished rural communities do not have the tax base from which to generate funding to cover the research needed to understand the unique factors that have an impact on the health of these residents or to establish, evaluate, and sustain programs and projects to address their needs and concerns. It is imperative that academic institutions, professional health care providers, political policy makers, and both private and public funding agencies acknowledge the high level of unmet needs in rural communities and then work collaboratively to address the behavioral health care needs of this large, but frequently overlooked, population.

There have been recent improvements and innovations that should be lauded—and expanded. Many academic institutions are beginning to include coverage of rural health and rural economic development in their training curriculum. Professional organizations have begun to establish rural agendas to help guide their actions and focus attention on the concerns of rural residents. Private foundations have begun to offer increasing funding options to various "grass roots" and professional groups interested in providing services for rural women and government sponsored agencies have begun to insist that residence, ethnicity, and age be among the variables addressed in proposals requesting research and/or service grant funds.

Similarly, support in the forms of grant funds and academic assistance should be provided for those groups, grass roots and/ or professional, which demonstrate a commitment to establishing sustainable, community-oriented programs and projects designed to identify and address the unmet needs of rural populations. Moreover, it is important to evaluate projects and programs to identify those that are most effective and then disseminate information about these successful interventions as widely as possible. Efforts to simplify the often intimidating process of applying for program development assistance and project funding should be continued. For example, current discussions among various state and federal grant agencies regarding the development of single "points of entry" for research and service delivery proposals are encouraging.

Future policies that are very likely to have a significant impact on the lives and overall health of rural women will include those related to parity for mental and physical health care, noting that the concept of "behavioral health" clearly demonstrates the importance of bridging the "mind/body gap," which has limited interdisciplinary collaboration among professionals. Policy makers should support programs and projects which address the broadest possible concerns, offer cost-effective solutions that can be sustained within the rural communities themselves, promote interdisciplinary cooperation, and provide specialized, culturally sensitive training opportunities, including both classroom and on-site internship experiences, for future professionals and paraprofessionals committed to serving rural patients.

REFERENCES

Agency for Health Care Policy and Research (1996). *Improving Health Care for Rural Populations Research in Action Fact Sheet* (AHCPR Publication No. 96-P040). Rockville, MD: Author.

Anahita, S. (1998). *Way out here: The unique situation of rural Iowa women in battering relationships.* Unpublished manuscript.

Anderson, J. E., Wilson, R., Doll, L., Jones, T. S., & Barker, P. (1999). Condom use and HIV risk behavior among U.S. adults: Data from a national survey. *Family Planning Perspectives, 31*(1), 24–28.

Beck, R. W., Jijon, C. R., & Edwards, J. B. (1996). The relationships among gender, perceived financial barriers to care, and health status in a rural population. *The Journal of Rural Health, 12*(3), 188–196.

Bergland, B. (1988). Rural mental health: Report of the National Action Commission on the mental health of rural Americans. *Journal of Rural Community Psychology, 9*(2), 29–39.

Bhatta, G. (2001). Of geese and ganders: Mainstreaming gender in the context of sustainable human development. *Journal of Gender Studies, 10*(1), 17–32.

Bushy, A. (1993). Rural women: Lifestyles and health status. *Nursing Clinics of North America, 28*(1), 187–197.

Centers for Disease Control. (1997). *Atlas reveals new mortality patterns for the United States.* Available at http://www.cdc.gov/od/oc/media/pressrel/deaths.htm

Crosby, R. A., Yarber, W. L., DiClemente, R. J., Wingood, G. M., & Meyerson, B. (2002). HIV-associated histories, perceptions, and practices among low-income African American women: Does rural residence matter? *American Journal of Public Health, 92*(4), 655–659.

Donnermeyer, F. (1995). Crime and violence in rural communities. In S. M. Blaser, J. Blaser, & K. Pantoja (Eds.), *Perspectives on violence and substance use in rural America,*. Oakbrook, IL: North Central Regional Educational Laboratory.

Duelberg, S. I. (1992). Preventive health behavior among Black and White women in urban and rural areas. *Social Sciences Medicine, 34*(2), 191–198.

Ford, D. H., & Lerner, R. M. (1992). *Developmental systems theory: An integrative approach.* Newbury Park, CA: Sage.

Frenzen, P. D., & Butler, M. A. (1997). Birth to unmarried mothers is rising faster in rural areas. *Rural Conditions and Trends, 8*(2), 66–69.

Gallagher, E., & Delworth, U. (1993). The third shift: Juggling employment, family, and the farm. *Journal of Rural Community Psychology, 12*(2), 21–36.

Glasgow, N., Holden, L., McLaughlin, P., & Rowles, R. (1993). Poverty among rural elders: Trends, context and directions for policy. *Journal of Applied Gerontology. 12*(3), 302–319.

Greenberg, M. R., Carey, G. W., & Popper, F. J. (1987). Violent death, violent states, and American youth. *Public Interest, 87,* 38–48.

Grieshop, J. I., Villanueva, N. E., & Stiles, M. C. (1994). Wash day blues: Second-hand exposure to agricultural chemicals. *The Journal of Rural Health, 10*(4), 247–257.

Khojasteh, A., Westhoff, D., Hackman, A., & Stone, J. (1999). *Patient viewpoints on mastectomy (M) versus lumpectomy (L) for breast cancer (BC)—A survey from the rural area.* Jefferson City, IA: Capitol Comprehensive Cancer Care Clinic/St. Mary Health Center.

McDuffie, H. H. (1994). Women at work: Agriculture and pesticides. *Journal of Occupational Medicine, 36*(11), 1240–1246.

Miller, K. (2003). Persistent Poverty in Rural America. *Perspectives on Poverty, Policy, and Place, 1*(1), 6–9.

Meadows, L. M., Thurston, W. E., & Berenson, C. A. (2001). Health promotion and preventive measures: Interpreting messages at midlife. *Qualitative Health Research, 11*(4), 450–463.

Mulder, P. L., & Chang, A. (1997). Domestic violence in rural communities: A literature review and discussion. *Journal of Rural Community Psychology, E1*(1). Retrieved October 4, 2004 from www.marshall.edu/jrcp/vole1/vol_e1_1/vole1no1.html

National Advisory Committee on Rural Health. (1993). *Sixth annual report on rural health.* Rockville, MD: U.S. Department of Health and Human Services.

National Center for Injury Prevention and Control. (1998). *Homicide and suicide among Native Americans, 1979–1992: Violence Surveillance Summary Series, No. 2.* Available at http://www.cdc.gov/ncipc/pub-res/natam.htm

National Rural Health Association. (1997). *HIV/AIDS in Rural America: An Issue Paper Prepared by the National Rural Health Association.* Baltimore, MD: Office of Research Development.

Rennison, C. M., & Welchans, S. (2000). *Intimate Partner Violence.* Washington, DC: Department of Justice, Bureau of Justice Statistics.

Rojewski, J. W., Wicklein, R. C., & Schell, J. W. (1995). Effects of gender and academic-risk behavior on the career maturity of rural youth. *Journal of Research in Rural Education, 11*(2), 1.

Rost, K., Williams, C., Wherry, J., & Smith, G. R., Jr. (1995). The process and outcomes of care for major depression in rural family practice settings. *The Journal of Rural Health, 11*(2), 114–121.

Schwenk, F. N. (1994). Income and consumer expenditures of rural elders. *Family Economics Review, 7*(3), 20–27.

Seccombe, K. (1995). Health insurance coverage and use of services among low-income elders: Does residence influence the relationship? *Journal of Rural Health, 11*(2), 86–97.

Seekins, T., Innes, B., & Maxon, N. (1998). *An Update on the Demography of Disability*. Missoula, MT: University of Montana, Rural Institute on Disabilities.

United States Congress Office of Technology Assessment. (1990). *Health care in rural America* (OTA-H-434). Washington, DC: United States Government Printing Office.

U.S. Congress, Office of Technology Assessment. (1990, September). *Health care in rural America* (OTA-H-434). Washington, DC: U.S. Government Printing Office.

U.S. Department of Agriculture. (2000). *Rural Income, Poverty, and Welfare: Rural Poverty*. Retrieved October 17, 2003 from http://ers.usda.gov/Briefing/income povertywelfare/RuralIncome/

U.S. Department of Agriculture. (1998). *Metro and nonmetro income data based on census information.* Available at http://www.usda.gov/news/pubs/fbook 98/ch4e.htm

U.S. Department of Agriculture. (1997). *Census of agriculture.* Washington, DC: Government Printing Office.

Van Hightower, N., & Dorsey, A. (2001). Reaching the hard to reach: Innovative responses to domestic violence. *Texas Journal of Rural Public Health, 29*(2), 30–41.

Van Hook, M. P. (1996). Challenges to identifying and treating women with depression in rural primary care. *Social Work in Health Care, 23*(3), 73–92.

Wagenfeld, M. O., Murray, J. D., Mohatt, D. F., & DeBruyn, J. C. (1993). *Mental health and rural America: 1980–1993*. Washington, DC: Office of Rural Health Policy.

Chapter 2

Policy Issues Affecting the Success of a Rural Women's Health Agenda

Kathleen M. McNamara

While it is encouraging that a book that focuses on linking the mental, behavioral, and physical health of rural women has been published, the policy issues which remain to be addressed in order to support a successful rural women's health agenda are significant.

In reviewing available health data, it is very discouraging to see the same discrepancies between metropolitan and rural populations cited in the health literature continue relatively unchanged over the past decade, especially for behavioral and mental health areas. The statistics reported in advocacy and policy documents are generally in the same direction: equal or higher prevalence and/or incidence among rural populations, with fewer resources in rural settings to address the problems. For rural women, as documented in other chapters of this book, the issues are even more challenging, in good part by virtue of their *de facto* roles in the fabric of rural culture.

Having reviewed the challenges and the socioeconomic and sociocultural stressors faced by rural women as presented by Mulder and Lambert (this volume), the question to be answered now is what will make the next decade any different? What are the policy issues which bear on improving the status of behavioral and mental health for rural populations? What policy changes hold more import for rural women independent of the overall rural population? This chapter will present a framework to begin to look for the answers.

The following areas pertinent to health care and health care delivery will serve as the structure for this discussion: availability, distribution, accessibility, effectiveness, and permanence of rural health professions (National Rural Health Association, 1992). The reader is cautioned that these categories are not mutually exclusive, and policy changes (or lack thereof) in one area may have impact on other areas.

AVAILABILITY OF SERVICES AND TRAINED PROVIDERS

Rural communities comprise half of the health professional shortage areas (HPSA) in the United States (Health Resources and Services Administration, 2003). In one survey, of the 55% of the counties across the nation with no psychologist, social worker or psychiatrist, all were rural counties (National Advisory Committee on Rural Health, 1993). HRSA attempted to address this lack of available providers by changing the label used to designate such areas from "psychiatric" to "mental health" professional shortage areas (MHPSA). With this designation, disciplines other than psychiatry could be included in federal programs relying on this designation. Access by rural areas to additional funds for providers and other resources was enhanced. While the potential to increase the overall number of available providers in rural areas is significant, for rural women the import of this policy decision is even more significant. In rural communities, where stigmatization is great, traditional medical models of service delivery for behavioral and mental health services have been limiting. The wider array of providers, with service delivery models not based on the medical model, should increase the probability that needed behavioral and mental health services, such as outreach services, will be available and will be utilized. The non-traditional service delivery models are more likely to be consumer-focused, guided by community input, and linked with other community-based services. These are the attributes that the National Rural

Health Association (NRHA, 1992) associates with a successful rural health system.

Meanwhile, the contributions of a federal program, the National Health Service Corps (NHSC), in adjusting the inequities of available health care between rural areas and metropolitan settings should be noted. The NHSC (U.S. Department of Health and Human Services, 2003) was created to "ensure an adequate supply of trained health professionals by assisting the repayment of qualifying educational loans in return for service to populations located in selected health professional shortage areas. . . . " However, inequities remain within that program, thus perpetuating the difficulty in providing behavioral and mental health services to rural communities. For example, of the 677 new and continuing loan repayment award recipients in 2002, 60 percent worked as primary health care providers, while only 21 percent worked as behavioral health care providers (U.S. Department of Health and Human Services, 2003a). While the existence of the NHSC clearly is to the advantage of rural communities, the current implementation is not serving rural women as well as it could. If there were a shift in the underlying policy from a segregation of physical health and behavioral health to an integration of behavioral health with primary care, available health professionals would be augmented. Those providing behavioral and mental health services through the NHSC would share equally in the awards, but would be expected to function differently, and even in different settings from what has been traditionally the case (i.e., Community Health Centers, not Community Mental Health Centers). Once an *integrated behavioral health care agenda* is adopted, providers who are better prepared to address the unique behavioral health needs of rural women could be identified.

Another federal program, the Quentin N. Burdick Program for Rural Health Interdisciplinary Training (Health Resources and Services Administration, 2003), addresses shortages of health professionals in rural areas in a very different manner. The program emphasizes interdisciplinary training projects, preparing health care professionals by training them in settings where persons of different disciplines work together. In addition, the program offers clinical training experiences in rural health care settings. Thus, the innovative concepts which support the program not only lean toward an integrated health care model requiring the development of new types of training, they also incorporate the rural setting as a necessary site for the training. This model for health professions training is more conducive to providing behavioral health care in a manner congruent with the rural lifestyle.

Along with considering new teaching and training strategies, it is important that other governmental programs which support training of rural health professionals be considered as underlying policy is reviewed. The Area Health Education Centers (AHECs) are one of the important programs in this category. AHECs are charged with focusing on community-based training of primary care providers, emphasizing "educational system incentives to attract and retain health care personnel in scarcity areas," and ultimately improving health care in underserved areas (Health Resources and Services Administration, 1996). How effective have the AHECs been in meeting this mandate? As was noted at the beginning of this chapter, the statistics and comments about discrepancies and inequities in rural health have not changed significantly over the past decade. There is no evidence that the AHECs fall outside of this norm. If one looks at policy decisions, perhaps something needs to be done differently, and the 2003 Congress considered one alternative. Since their creation, AHECs have been established through cooperative agreements *only with schools of medicine or osteopathy*. The 2003 legislation provides for cooperative agreements with schools of nursing in certain situations. There is no reason not to expand this access to an even broader array of training programs and institutions, such as schools of professional psychology or schools of social work, which focus more specifically on behavioral and mental health training. The continual reliance on a philosophy of training and service delivery primarily based on a traditional medical model does not seem to have been effective in leveling the differences. While not advocating for eliminating the involvement of medical schools, perhaps what is necessary is what Senator Ron Wyden (D-Ore), in addressing the problem of aging and the shortage of trained providers (U.S. Senate, Senate Special Committee on Aging, 2003) referred to as "nothing short of a revolution" in the national medical education system. The report of the Substance Abuse and Mental Health Services Administration's (SAMHSA) work group to address Mental Health Providers in Rural and Isolated Areas (U.S. Department of Health and Human Services, 1997) provided several recommendations which clearly speak to this revolution relative to behavioral and mental health shortages. The work group directed that the mental health professions "should actively encourage innovative training strategies . . . explicitly targeted at expanding the competencies required to practice effectively in rural settings," and that "training programs should make concerted efforts to recruit qualified applicants from rural areas who are more likely to practice in rural locations after graduation." The work group elaborated upon the need for interdisciplinary collaboration to "enhance the supply" and "improve consumer access" to providers of mental health care. The members of that group further indicated that "training programs and credentialing bodies should identify which of their current practices create barriers . . . and work toward removing these impediments."

Distribution of Providers

While policy changes in our educational programs may change the availability of well-trained behavioral and mental health providers for rural practice, what is to be done to recruit and retain them in needed areas? At a very basic level, relevant statistics on these provider groups were not readily accessible on various federal agency Web sites or in official reports and documents. Consequently, a starting point would be a policy shift requiring the tracking of these providers, since knowing their number and location is as important as knowing about the primary care physicians in any HPSA (statistics which are readily available). Implicit in this decision would be a shift in the balance of attention given to behavioral health by entities such as the Office of Rural Health Policy (Health Resources and Services Administration, 2003a) at the federal level, and each of the Offices of Rural Health at the State level. Specifically acknowledging behavioral and mental health through assigning in-house staff with responsibility for this program area, requiring representation of behavioral health experts on advisory boards, and including specific initiatives in strategic plans would signal to others that the value given to linking behavioral, mental and physical health has changed. While these changes address broadly the emphasis on behavioral and mental health in rural communities, additional advocacy can lead to more focused attention on specific segments of the population, such as rural women. Just as infant mortality, diabetes, or teen pregnancy fall out of primary care agendas, the unique behavioral and mental health needs of rural women can become a designated initiative. The impact of this policy change would come full circle with the emphasis on actually delivering the needed services, since the demand for an adequate supply of providers at the sites of intervention should increase.

There are a number of locations within the federal government where policy related to the distribution of behavioral and mental health care providers can be influenced. The HRSA Bureau of Health Professions Web site (hhtp://bhpr.hrsa.gov) explicitly states that one of its major goals is to improve access to quality health care through *appropriate distribution* of the health professions workforce (italics added). Similarly, within the mission of the Office of Rural Health Policy (Health Resources and Services Administration, 2003) is a charge to evaluate the ability of rural areas to attract and retain physicians and other health professionals. In a March, 1992 letter to then Secretary of Health and Human Services, Louis W. Sullivan, Senator Daniel Inouye addressed issues of distribution, stating "federal health programs by their very design discourage the creative use of nonphysician mental and allied health professionals" (personal communication, April 1, 1992). He urged "better alignment" of mental and behavioral health care needs and the resources to meet them "through appropriate federal policies." The HRSA Bureau of Health Professions (U.S. Department of Health and Human Services, 2003) notes that at least 34 federal programs depend on the HPSA designation to determine eligibility or to denote a funding preference. The potential for securing resources specifically tagged for rural women's initiatives through these and other federal programs is uncharted. Not only could the systematic use of the HPSA/MHPSA designation specifically guide the funding of rural women's behavioral health initiatives, but incentives for mental health professionals to practice and remain in shortage areas also could be inherent in the initiatives.

In the 2003 federal legislation referred to as the Medicare Prescription Drug and Modernization Act, members of a group referred to as the Senate Rural Caucus have demonstrated the effectiveness of a strong voice on behalf of rural communities. That legislation contained "rural amendments," which proposed, among other changes, that physicians practicing in primary or specialty care scarcity counties would be given an additional 5 percent Medicare bonus payment. Those who share the concern for rural women's behavioral and mental health must partner with members of this Congressional Rural Caucus to effect policies and influence decisionmakers in a way that will advance the rural women's agenda.

Accessibility of Services and Providers

Reviewing the listings for rural health on the HRSA Web site yields many entries for race, ethnicity, and minority groups, but references for rural women are nonexistent. Yet, the Web site clearly states that one segment of HRSA, the Bureau of Health Professions Programs, is to assure access to quality health care professionals *in all geographic areas* and *to all segments of society* (italics added). The site describes the current goals: (1) improve access to quality health care through appropriate preparation, composition, and distribution of the health professions workforce, and (2) improve access to a diverse and culturally competent and sensitive health professions workforce (U.S. Department of Health and Human Services, 2003). The lack of references to women and rural women speaks volumes about the inconsistency between the stated goals and the current state of the implementation of the mission and goals.

One element, which might help to address such an inconsistency, would be the existence of an appropriate interdisciplinary curriculum focused on the needs of rural women, similar to the full scope Interdisciplinary Rural Curriculum promulgated by the American Psychological Association (APA, 1995). Such an initiative, combined with strategies already discussed in other sections, could lead to improved access for rural women to the appropriately trained and sensitive health professions workforce that HRSA purports to be seeking. The Quentin N. Burdick Rural Program for Interdisciplinary Training has provided grants whose purpose was to demonstrate and evaluate "methods and models that improve access to cost effective, comprehensive health care" (Health Resources and Services Administration, 2003). The outcome of such projects needs to be disseminated as widely as possible, and their relevance for delivery of services to rural women needs to be evaluated.

The National Association for Rural Mental Health (NARMH, 2002) also addressed access issues, stating that "Community Health Centers should provide integrated mental health services especially in rural and frontier areas" and urged HRSA to work to "ensure that rural residents are able to access behavioral health services through their Community Health Centers."

Presently, the Department of Agriculture has the mandate to coordinate federal rural development efforts, and the portfolio consists of over 800 programs administered by various federal departments (Rural Policy Research Institute, 2003). Is it any wonder that the attention given to rural women's needs is sparse to nonexistent? The Rural Policy Research Institute (RUPRI) has called for considering a federal Department of Rural Affairs, similar to what Texas has done. If such a development were to occur, the probability becomes greater that a rural women's behavioral health agenda would be carved out. However, there still remains no guarantee that behavioral health would have equal footing. Since rural residents typically are more likely to be underinsured or uninsured, unless this basic issue is addressed, equal access to behavioral and mental health services will still remain out of reach. Even with third-party coverage, it is not unusual for disparities to exist in coverage for behavioral health. While support of federal and state mental health parity legislation is one avenue for addressing this discrimination, efforts that improve linkages and promote full integration of behavioral health with primary care would break down the artificial separation of physical and mental health. Support for innovative service delivery models that encourage interventions around natural support networks also would facilitate access. This would be especially true for rural women, given the sociocultural barriers discussed by other authors in an earlier chapter.

Effectiveness

A formal research agenda can be developed around the measurement of effectiveness, and the NRHA (1999) included in its issue paper on mental health in rural America a specific section on rural mental health services research. The NRHA urged HRSA, as well as the National Institutes of Mental Health (NIMH) and SAMSHA to provide the leadership and funding to accomplish that agenda. The knowledge gaps to which that issue paper referred continue today, but the National Institute of Mental Health (2003) now has an Office of Rural Mental Health Research (ORMHR), which "directs, plans, coordinates, and supports research activities and information dissemination on conditions unique to those living in rural areas, including research on the delivery of mental health services in such areas." Closer alliances with academic institutions with particular interest in rural initiatives are needed to promote the agenda of this office, and to tailor aspects of the funding priorities to rural women's behavioral health. Support in the forms of grant funds and academic assistance should be provided for those which demonstrate a commitment to establishing sustainable community oriented programs and carrying out projects identifying and tackling the unmet needs of rural populations. Evaluating projects and programs, identifying those which are most effective, and then widely disseminating information about successful interventions can contribute necessary supporting materials to effect policy changes.

Individual rural providers, typically "generalists," must have access to knowledge which will expand their "specialist" skills if they are to be effective in the delivery of needed services. Health centers, professional organizations, and other support networks need adequate funding to access the training to increase these skills. In this era of distance learning and telehealth applications, geographic distance should not be a barrier for providers seeking to improve the effectiveness of their interventions. While addressing funding for the Bureau of Health Professions, members of the U.S. Senate committee reviewing the legislation explicitly stated that they expected expanded support for telehealth initiatives for providing distance education and training for professions serving the rural areas. The Rural Mental Health Provider Work Group addressed this as well, stating that "creative applications of information technology (e.g., telecommunications) that are aimed at reducing barriers to accessing mental health services in rural areas and sound evaluations of their effectiveness should be promoted" (U.S. Department of Health and Human Services, 1997). NARMH (2002) went further and placed the responsibility with HRSA and SAMHSA for directing necessary funding and technical assistance to "programs and agencies that want to attempt effective coordination and integration" of behavioral health and primary care in rural areas.

While the above discussion focuses on *what can be done*, it also is important to indicate *what should not be done*. To the extent that other governmental decisions do not consider the nuances of implementing rules or regulations in rural settings, they may be contributing to mental health problems. The welfare reform back-to-work initiative is an example. While implementation may be relatively streamlined in metropolitan areas with available transportation, child care, and access to a range of jobs with varying skill levels, it is not so easily executed in rural communities where the population is quite spread out and the jobs are distant from the home, where no public transportation exists, the family has one vehicle, and no child-care services are readily available. Unless the various governmental agencies begin to consider the interpretation of regulations in light of rural factors, an exacerbation of stressors can be anticipated. The very stressors that mental and behavioral health services are trying to eliminate are now iatrogenic! In its Policy and Action Agenda, NARMH (2002) recommended that SAMHSA ensure that "any group . . . that develops practice guidelines or standards for behavioral health interventions/practice include rural representation and ensure that the guidelines be reviewed for rural applicability and feasibility. . . . " This same report calls for SAMHSA to work with grant programs to publish a "best/promising practices report," and identify "lessons learned." While these admonitions begin to raise the consciousness of policymakers about the differences between metropolitan and rural communities, the unique behavioral and mental health needs of rural women must be considered with the same awareness that there are differences that justify such a separate analysis.

Permanence

The problem of recruiting and retaining behavioral health providers in rural areas has no simple solution, and the focus of such efforts to date may have been too limited. Rather than looking for incentives to keep providers once they are located in the rural setting, an alternative approach could start with asking what needs to be done to attract rural residents into the health professions workforce, and how is this facilitated? A significant finding with direct bearing on this question was reported by the Bureau of Health Professions (U.S. Department of Health and Human Services, 1990). Fewer than 17% of nonphysician health personnel resided in nonmetropolitan communities, whereas at the time, 23% of the United States population did. But, more telling, was the fact that fewer than 3% of nonmetropolitan counties had accredited training programs for nonphysician health professionals, and less than 13% of the training programs for nonphysicians were located in nonmetropolitan areas. The scarcity of training sites would severely limit access for those entering the rural labor force who might seek training and employment in health careers. While more current data were not found to cover the past decade, if the situation is not significantly different, clearly the augmentation of telehealth initiatives and distance learning opportunities for rural settings must be a priority. The Bureau of Health Professions would be a logical federal site for overseeing such a development of resources, but partnership with the state Offices of Rural Health would seem essential to success. Once individuals already residing in rural settings become part of the health care workforce in those same settings, issues around the permanence of the providers in a community can be taken from the negative side of the equation and placed on the positive side. This workforce has the additional advantage of possessing a unique understanding of what it means to be living in a rural environment and to need mental health assistance. Further, this workforce could easily comprise rural women, who know firsthand the struggles and barriers to accessing that assistance. In addition, as recommended by the Rural Mental Health Provider Work Group, the inclusion of "natural helpers and traditional healers found in rural cultures" would increase the resources coming from the already permanent members of the community.

While providers living and working in the community is the ideal, can an assimilation occur with nearly equal acceptance for itinerant providers from surrounding communities? Will innovative applications of telehealth eventually overcome the "distance" element in the technology, and the providers achieve acceptance as "members" of the community? What innovations will facilitate the permanence of services without revisiting the "town-gown" split often seen with the intrusion of medical schools into local medical centers? And, if solutions are found in any of these areas, will the perception and acceptance be the same among the community of rural women with behavioral and mental health care needs as it might be among the broader rural community? There is no simple solution, but there must be a research and educational agenda that considers the psychological, social, and cultural factors underlying the definition of "permanence."

Once a workforce is in place, what factors influence the permanency of providers or programs? As implied in earlier comments, federal and state regulations can promote fractioning rather than integration of services. Without attention to the rural applicability and nuances in implementation of regulations and standards, personal and financial costs become burdensome and create disincentives, with a higher likelihood that there will be a negative outcome for rural women.

To the extent that reimbursement and funding mechanisms or requirements are complicated, restrictive, and/or time-consuming, providers and programs are less likely to remain in rural and frontier areas. The NARMH (2002) report called for a National Rural Behavioral Health Technical Assistance Center/Program to assist with practice and management issues. Further, the report called for a realistic assessment of the cost of delivering services in rural areas that would serve as the basis for "cost-based reimbursement." The U.S. Department of Health and Human Services (1997) provider work group recommended that mental health providers in rural areas be allowed to "deliver and be reimbursed for the full range of services for which they have the appropriate skills and competencies." Until the nonphysician health care workforce no longer has unnecessary limitations imposed on their scope of practice and is able to exercise their skills to meet the demands they perceive in the health care arena, the type of role and work satisfaction that can serve as a basis for permanence will always be at risk.

The recent emphasis on information technology (IT) is not lost on those addressing rural and frontier behavioral and mental health needs (National Association for Rural Mental Health, 2002; National Rural Health Association, 1999; U.S. Department of Health and Human Services, 1997). While IT is certainly applicable to innovations in the delivery of clinical services, it also holds significant potential for addressing underlying issues associated with problems in recruitment and retention of well-trained providers. Access to college courses, advanced professional continuing education, and direct communication with peers and consultation with specialists is now possible. The isolation and concerns about remaining abreast of current information, which once were major elements in the loss of providers from rural communities, no longer need to be contributing factors. The wealth of available information on the Internet, and the ease of access, can bring rural providers into the mainstream with relative ease. Where the database is not well developed (e.g., rural women and behavioral health), practitioner networks can be established across the nation to share "promising practices" and allow the database to evolve. Obviously, if rural communities have not experienced the expansion of the infrastructure to keep up with technological advances, they are once again at a disadvantage relative to their metropolitan counterparts. This is simply not acceptable, and certainly not consistent with the expectations of the Congressional Rural Caucus, with whom a close partnership is encouraged.

As we conclude this chapter, an excerpt from *Healthy People 2010* seems especially relevant: "Over the years, it has become clear that individual health is closely linked to community health—the health of the community and environment in which the individuals live, work, and play. Likewise, community health is profoundly affected by the collective behaviors, attitudes, and beliefs of everyone who lives in that community" (U.S. Department of Health and Human Services, 2000). The very fabric of rural society and its expectations for the roles rural women must assume are intertwined with the behavioral and mental health care needs of rural women and their families, and with the implicit assumptions which drive the public policies addressing those needs.

REFERENCES

American Psychological Association (1995). *Caring for the rural community: An interdisciplinary curriculum.* Washington, DC: Author.

Health Resources and Services Administration (1996). *Fact sheet: Area health education centers.* Bureau of Health Professions, Department of Health and Human Services. Washington, DC: Author.

Health Resources and Services Administration (2003). *The Quentin N. Burdick Rural Program for Interdisciplinary Training.* Retrieved September 10, 2003, from http://bhpr.hrsa.gov/shortage

Health Resources and Services Administration (2003a). *Description, Office of Rural Health Policy.* Retrieved September 10, 2003, from http://www.rural health.hrsa.gov

National Advisory Committee on Rural Health (1993). *Sixth annual report on rural health*. Rockville, MD: U.S. Department of Health and Human Services.

National Association for Rural Mental Health (2002). *Rural mental and behavioral health policy and action agenda*. St. Cloud, MN: Author.

National Institutes of Mental Health (2003). *Description, Office of Rural Mental Health Research*. Retrieved September 9, 2003, from www.nimh.nih.gov/ormhr

National Rural Health Association (1992). *Study of Models to Meet Rural Health Needs Through Mobilization of Health Professions Education and Services Resources: A Rural Health Agenda for the Future*. Report prepared under contract for the Bureau of Health Professions, Health Resources and Services Administration, Rockville, Maryland.

National Rural Health Association (1999). *Mental Health in Rural America: An Issue Paper*. Kansas City, Missouri.

Rural Policy Research Institute (2003). *Editorial: What's Good for Texas*. Retrieved September 9, 2003, from http://www.rupri.org

U.S. Department of Health and Human Services. (1990). *Rural Health Professions Facts: Supply and Distribution of Health Professions in Rural America*, Health Resources and Services Administration, Bureau of Health Professions, Washington, D.C..

U.S. Department of Health and Human Services (1997). *Mental Health Providers in Rural and Isolated Areas, Final Report of the Ad Hoc Rural Mental Health Provider Work Group*, Substance Abuse and Mental Health Services Administration, Washington, D.C.

U.S. Department of Health and Human Services (2000). *Healthy People 2010: Understanding and improving health*. Washington, DC: Author.

U.S. Department of Health and Human Services (2003). *Health Professions Shortage Areas*. Bureau of Health Professions, HRSA. Retrieved September 10, 2003, from http://bhpr.hrsa.gov/shortage

U.S. Department of Health and Human Services (2003a). National Health Service Corps. Retrieved September 10, 2003, from http://nhsc.bhpr.hrsa.gov

U.S. Senate, Special Committee on Aging (2003, May). *Ageism in the health care system: Shortshrifting seniors?* Washington, DC: U.S. Government Printing Office.

Chapter 3

Differences in Mental Health Indicators and Psychotropic Drug Use Between Rural and Nonrural Older Women

Carol Hancock Gold, Kelli L. Dominick, Frank M. Ahern, and Debra A. Heller

Older women face chronic medical conditions and life circumstances that can have adverse effects on their mental health. Diseases such as diabetes and heart disease have been associated with an increase in depressive symptoms (Fried & Wallace, 1992). Disability associated with chronic illness and Activities of Daily Living (ADL) impairments are associated with an increase in emotional and psychosomatic distress (Revicki & Mitchell, 1990). Resources for home health services in the rural environment are limited, as compared with more populated urban areas (Esposito, 1994). Many older women take on the role of caregivers to their husbands and others, and caregiver stress has been shown to lead to mental health

The authors would like to thank PACE for providing the data used in this study. This research was funded by a cooperative agreement (TS213) from the Centers for Disease Control and Prevention (CDC) with the Association of Teachers of Preventive Medicine.

45

problems such as depression, anxiety, and sleep difficulties, as well as increased psychotropic drug use (Horsley, Barrow, Gent, & Astbury, 1998; Mort, Gaspar, Juffer, & Kovarna, 1996). In a study of elderly caregivers, a greater number of those who were rural considered themselves to be in poor or fair health than those in the general population (Sanford & Townsend-Rocchiccioli, 2004). Some rural women have been caregivers for many years because of permanently disabling injuries experienced by their farmer husbands (Reed & Claunch, 2002). With age, many older women become widowed and experience loneliness and isolation (Gale, 1993), especially in the presence of chronic diseases that limit their functioning. Resulting mental health problems can be exacerbated by the conditions of rural isolation (Russell, Cutrona, de la Mora, & Wallace, 1997).

Prior research suggests underutilization of mental health services and psychotropic medication by rural older adults (Fox, Blank, Berman, & Rovnyak, 1999; Maiden & Peterson, 2002; Ganguli, Mulsant, Richards, Stoehr, & Mendelsohn, 1997). Contributing factors may include negative attitudes toward mental health services (Maiden & Peterson, 2002), lack of mental health providers (Rost, Fortney, Zhang, Smith, & Smith, 1999), burnout of rural health providers (Thommasen, Lavanchy, Connelly, Berkowitz, & Grzybowski, 2001), and difficulty getting to a provider (Fortney, Rost, Zhang, & Warren, 1999). The study by Fox and colleagues (1999) found a lack of acknowledgement of the need for help among rural residents, even among those who were identified (and notified) as having mental health problems that should be treated. Research has also found that, in light of the many other pressing needs for health care in rural settings, residents of rural communities placed a lesser value on access to mental health services (Watts et al., 1999).

Most studies that have examined rural/urban differences in mental health problems and treatment have looked at both older men and women. A recent study found that rural location predicted an increased likelihood of antidepressant and hypnotic/anxiolytic prescriptions among elderly persons (Craig et al., 2003). Another research study found that receiving health care in a metropolitan area decreased the likelihood of potentially inappropriate prescriptions to the ambulatory elderly (Mort & Aparasu, 2000). In a previous study, findings suggested underutilization of antidepressant drugs in rural older adults (Ganguli, Mulsant, Richards, Stoehr, & Mendelsohn, 1997).

Little research has focused on rural/urban differences in indicators of mental health problems and treatment among older women. The goal of this study was to examine differences between rural and urban older women in: (1) self-reported indicators of mental health problems; (2) physician visits with a diagnosis for depression or anxiety; and (3) psychotropic prescription drug use.

METHODS

Participants

The sample consisted of 28,561 women who were enrolled in the Pennsylvania Pharmaceutical Assistance Contract for the Elderly (PACE) program in 1997. PACE is a state program that helps to pay for prescription medications for Pennsylvanians age 65 and older whose annual income does not exceed $20,200, if married, or $17,000, if single. The program covers all prescription drugs as well as insulin syringes and needles; enrollees pay a small copayment (ranging from $6 to $15) for each prescription. Depending on their annual income, PACE cardholders are required to reapply for coverage either annually or biannually. In 1997, 172,647 printed surveys based on the Centers for Disease Control and Prevention's (CDC) Health-Related Quality of Life (HRQOL) module were included with PACE applications mailed to cardholders who were scheduled to renew their coverage. Among 144,819 cardholders who returned their renewal application to PACE, a total of 83,471 also returned a completed survey, yielding a survey response rate of 58%. Respondents and nonrespondents were similar with respect to characteristics including age, gender, race, residential status, marital status, and annual income.

Medicare eligibility data, Part A (hospitalization data), and Part B (physician/supplier) data files were provided by the Centers for Medicare and Medicaid Services, who performed data linkage and record extraction for the sample of survey respondents. The analyses described here focus on outpatient physician visit data contained in the Medicare Part B files. Some survey respondents were not eligible for Medicare benefits for the entire year following the survey completion, or were members of an HMO that processed their Medicare claims for at least part of that year. Since complete Medicare data were not available for these individuals, they were excluded from this study.

Demographic information for survey respondents was obtained from the PACE cardholder files, including the county of residence, which enabled rural/urban classification. The United States Department of Agriculture's Rural-Urban Continuum Codes classification scheme was used to categorize counties in Pennsylvania by degree of urbanization and nearness to a metropolitan area (Rural Policy Research Institute, 1999). Counties designated as metropolitan in this scheme were classified as urban, and counties designated as nonmetropolitan were classified as rural. Using this classification system, we categorized the study sample of 28,561 women as urban (N = 22,400) or rural (N = 6,161). The mean age of the sample was 79.4 years old, with a range of 65 to 104 years of age. The mean annual income in the year preceding the survey was $10,689. The majority of respondents were white (94%); living in the community, i.e., not in nursing homes, personal care homes, or assisted living facilities (96.3%); and widowed, divorced, single, or not living with spouse (94%).

Measures

Self-Reported Mental Health Indicators

All participants had completed the CDC HRQOL module. This was a self-administered, mail-based survey that asked participants to report on their physical and mental health. The three questions examined in the current study as mental health indicators were:

1. Now thinking about your mental health, which includes stress, depression, and problems with emotions, for how many days during the past 30 days was your **mental health not good**? (mentally unhealthy days)

2. During the past 30 days, for about how many days have you felt **sad, blue, or depressed**? (depressed mood days)

3. During the past 30 days, for about how many days have you felt **worried, tense, or anxious**? (anxiety days)

Physician Visits with Codes for Depression and Anxiety

Medicare Part B files were used to generate dichotomous variables regarding any physician visit with a primary or secondary ICD-9 (1998) code of major depression (296.2 and 296.3), minor depression (300.4), or anxiety (300.0). These variables were assessed for a one-year period following the completion date of the HRQOL survey for each subject.

Psychotropic Prescription Drug Use

Use of antidepressants and anxiolytics during the year following the completion of the HRQOL survey were assessed from PACE claims history files for each person in the study. Using a proprietary database, the Medi-Span Master Drug Database®, all prescriptions filled by participants for antidepressants and anxiolytics were identified (Generic Product Indicator Codes of 58 and 57, respectively). We examined whether or not subjects filled a prescription for any antidepressant or anxiolytic during the study period, as well as use of specific types of antidepressants and anxiolytics. Dichotomous variables indicating use of any antidepressant and anxiolytic were generated, as well as variables indicating use of specific types of antidepressants (selective serotonin reuptake inhibitors [SSRIs] and tricyclic antidepressants [TCAs]), and anxiolytics (buspirone and benzodiazepines).

Covariates

Multivariate analyses included demographic and health-related variables that may have affected self-reported mental health indicators, physician diagnoses of depression and anxiety, and the use of psychotropic medication. Demographic covariates included age, race (White/non-White), annual income, nursing home status, and marital status. For some analyses, examining physician visits and psychotropic drug use, the number of mentally unhealthy days, or the number of depressed mood days, were included in order to adjust for possible group differences in psychological health.

Statistical Analyses

Rural/urban differences in the means of the self-reported mental health measures were examined using t-tests. Multivariate regression analyses were used to examine rural/urban differences in these indicators while controlling for demographic factors. Chi-square tests examined rural/urban differences in all dichotomous variables (e.g., any physician visit with a major depression diagnosis, any use of an antidepressant, etc.). Multivariate logistic regression models were used to test for rural/urban differences in each dichotomous variable, adjusting for demographic factors and mental health-related covariates, such as number of depressed days or mentally unhealthy days in past 30 days.

RESULTS

Self-Reported Mental Health Indicators

Table 3.1 presents bivariate results on rural/urban differences in selected self-reported mental health measures. The results of t-tests indicated that, on average, urban women reported significantly more mentally unhealthy days in the previous 30 ($p = .005$), depressed mood ($p = .022$), and anxiety ($p = .016$) than did rural women. After adjusting for demographic factors, regression analyses confirmed that urban women reported significantly more mentally unhealthy days ($p < .05$) and anxiety days ($p < .05$); however, there was no longer a significant difference in number of depressed mood days for urban and rural women.

TABLE 3.1   Mean Number of Days in Past 30 and t-Test Results of Self-Reported Mental Health Indicators According to Rural/Urban Status

Self-reported mental health variable	Rural (N = 5,898)	Urban (N = 21,460)	p Value
Mentally unhealthy days [Means (SD)]	3.76 (8.4)	4.11 (8.7)	.005
Depressed mood days [Means (SD)]	4.76 (8.9)	5.07 (9.2)	.022
Anxiety days [Means (SD)]	5.63 (9.7)	5.98 (10.0)	.016

Physician Visits with Codes for Depression and Anxiety

Table 3.2 summarizes analyses of diagnoses for depression and anxiety during physician visits in the 12-month period following the survey. Rural women were less likely to have a physician visit involving a code for depression ($p < .001$), and specifically for major depression ($p < .001$). Even after adjusting for demographic factors and number of bad mental health days, rural women were less likely than urban women to have had a physician visit with a code for depression in general (odds ratio (OR) = 0.75; 95% CI: 0.63–0.89) or for major depression (OR = 0.67; 95% CI: 0.55–0.83). Thus, rural women were 25% less likely to have been diagnosed with depression, in general, and 33% less likely to have been diagnosed with major depression, than urban women, according to the Medicare records of physician visits. No significant differences were found between rural and urban women in the likelihood of having a physician visit with a code of minor depression or anxiety.

Since 14 or more days of depressed mood in 30 days can indicate possible clinical depression, we examined the subsample of women

TABLE 3.2 Diagnosis of Selected Mental Health Problems During Physician Visits in the 12-Month Follow-Up Period According to Rural/Urban Status: Bivariate and Multivariate Results

Type of diagnosis	% of Rural (N = 6,161)	% of Urban (N = 22,400)	p Value	Adjusted[1] OR for Rural	95% CI	p Value
Any depression	2.7	3.5	< .001	0.75	0.63–0.89	.001
Major depression	1.9	2.7	< .001	0.67	0.55–0.83	< .001
Minor depression	0.9	1.1	.358	0.90	0.67–1.21	.467
Anxiety	3.7	3.7	.865	0.99	0.85–1.16	.911

[1]Adjusted for age, race, income, nursing home status, marital status, and number of mentally unhealthy days.
Note: The c-statistic indicated a good model fit for all multivariate models.

who fell in that category. Logistic regression analyses were carried out, adjusting for demographic factors and number of depressed mood days (to control for the seriousness of the problem) of these women. Again, rural women who met this criterion were significantly less likely than urban women to have had a physician visit involving a code for major depression in the year following the survey (OR = 0.68; 95% CI: 0.49–0.93). In other words, among women who reported 14 or more days of depressed mood in 30 days, rural women were 32% less likely to receive a code for major depression from the physician than were urban women.

Psychotropic Prescription Drug Use

Table 3.3 presents information on respondents' psychotropic drug utilization in the 12 months following survey completion. In bivariate analyses, 17.0% of rural and 17.3% of urban women had filled a prescription for at least one antidepressant ($p = .625$), indicating no significant difference in this measure. However, urban women were significantly more likely to have been prescribed a SSRI (10.9% vs. 9.5%, $p = .002$), and rural women were more likely to have been prescribed a TCA (6.1% vs. 5.4%, $p = .033$). Rural women were also more likely to have filled a prescription for at least one anxiolytic (23.4% vs. 21.8%, $p = .005$), and, more specifically, benzodiazepines (20.3% vs. 19%, $p = .018$) and buspirone (1.9% vs. 1.5%, $p = .02$). Analyses that adjusted for demographic factors and number of mentally unhealthy days revealed the same significant findings with one exception: there was only a trend ($p = .09$) for the rural women regarding higher use of TCAs.

Additional analyses focused on only those women who had reported 14 or more depressed mood days in the past 30 days (not shown). In this subsample, 33.2% of rural women and 36.2% of urban women had filled a prescription for an antidepressant in the 12-month period following the survey ($p = .09$). Logistic regression analyses of these women showed that, adjusting for demographic factors and number of depressed mood days, there was some indication, although not significant ($p = .067$), that rural women were less likely to receive an antidepressant in the year following the HRQOL survey (OR = 0.86; 95% CI: 0.73–1.01). In other words, among this

TABLE 3.3 Use of Selected Psychotropic Drugs During the 12-Month Follow-Up Period According to Rural/Urban Status: Bivariate and Multivariate Results

Psychotropic Category	% of Rural (N = 6,161)	% of Urban (N = 22,400)	p Value	Adjusted[1] OR for Rural	95% CI	p Value
Any anti-depressant	17.0	17.3	0.625	0.99	0.91–1.07	.775
SSRI antide-pressant	9.5	10.9	0.002	0.88	0.79–0.97	.009
Tricyclic antide-pressant	6.1	5.4	0.033	1.11	0.98–1.26	.089
Any anxiolytic	23.4	21.8	0.005	1.10	1.02–1.18	.010
Benzodia-zepine	20.3	19.0	0.018	1.08	1.003–1.16	.040
Buspirone	1.9	1.5	0.020	1.32	1.06–1.64	.015

[1]Adjusted for age, race, income, nursing home status, marital status, and number of mentally unhealthy days.
Note: The c-statistic indicated a good model fit for all multivariate models.

group of women who had reported 14 or more depressed mood days in a month, rural women were 14% less likely to have filled a prescription for an antidepressant than were urban women.

Table 3.4 focuses on only those older women who had filled a prescription for an antidepressant in the 12-month follow-up period. In this sample, bivariate analyses showed that rural women were significantly more likely to have been prescribed a tricyclic antide-pressant (p < .01) than were urban women. Analyses that adjusted for demographic factors and number of depressed mood days found that among this selected sample, there was some indication, albeit nonsignificant (p = .0625), that rural women were approximately 15% more likely to have been prescribed a tricyclic antidepressant (OR = 1.15; 95% CI: 0.99–1.34) than were urban women.

TABLE 3.4   Tricyclic Antidepressant Use by Women Prescribed an Antidepressant During the 12-Month Follow-Up Period According to Rural/Urban Status: Bivariate and Multivariate Results

	% of Rural (N = 1,050)	% of Urban (N = 3,877)	p Value	Adjusted[1] OR for Rural	95% CI	p Value
Use of Tricyclic Antidepressant	35.8	31.2	.005	1.15	0.99– 1.34	.063

[1]Adjusted for age, race, income, nursing home status, marital status, and number of depressed mood days.
Note: The c-statistic indicated a good model fit for the multivariate model.

DISCUSSION

Linkage among three extensive datasets provided us with a clearer understanding of the rural/urban differences among older women in mental health indicators, physician visits involving codes for specific mental health problems, and use of selected prescription psychotropics. Several notable findings, discussed below, have been discovered in these analyses of rural and urban older women.

Urban women reported more days of anxiety in the past 30 days than did rural women, and yet rural women were significantly more likely to have filled a prescription for an anxiolytic in the 12-month follow-up period than were urban women. This finding persisted even after adjusting for demographic factors and number of mentally unhealthy days in the past 30 days. Nearly a quarter (23.4%) of the rural women and 21.8% of the urban women had filled a prescription for at least one anxiolytic in that period. Upon examining physician visit data, we found that there was no rural/urban difference in the percentage of older women who received a diagnosis code of anxiety in the 12-month follow-up period. Also, only 3.7% of rural and urban women had a physician visit with this diagnosis code during this one-year follow-up. Thus the large number of both rural and urban women receiving prescriptions for anxiolytics may have been diagnosed with anxiety in the previous year or earlier, with no follow-up diagnosis codes indicated in our 12-month period. It may be that the physicians are following up on these women, but not continuing to document the code. However it is important to emphasize that lack of surveillance of psychological disorders, with continued issuance of prescriptions for psychotropic medications, can lead to serious problems, particularly in the elderly.

It is also of interest that, despite the fact that multivariate regression analyses indicated no significant difference in self-reported number of depressed mood days for urban and rural women, rural women were significantly less likely to have a physician visit with a code for depression in the 12-month period following this self-report. This finding persisted in logistic regression analyses that adjusted for demographic factors and number of mentally unhealthy days. The latter covariate was included because of the importance of adjusting for possible group differences in psychological health. In other words, one cannot attribute fewer physician visits with codes for depression among rural older women to the possibility that they were psychologically healthier.

In order to examine this finding even more carefully, we conducted additional analyses for the subgroup of women who had reported 14 or more depressed mood days out of the past 30 days in the HRQOL study. Several authoritative sources speculate that this self-report measure would be a good indicator of diagnosable depression (Borawski, Wu, & Jia, 1998; Durch, Bailey, & Stoto, 1997). It also correlates with one of the Diagnostic and Statistical Manual of Mental Disorders (DSM-IV, 1994) criteria for depression, i.e., 2 weeks or more of depressed mood. Again, we found that rural women were significantly less likely to have had a physician visit with a code for depression. In these analyses we adjusted for demographic factors and for the number of depressed mood days reported. Again, by including the latter covariate, we feel confident that the finding that these rural women had significantly fewer physician visits with a code for depression cannot be attributed to a possible group difference in number of depressed mood days.

The finding that among older women who reported a fairly severe level of depressed mood (14+ days in past 30), rural women were less likely than urban women to have had a physician visit with a depression code during the 12-month follow-up is not surprising in light of prior findings related to underutilization of mental health services by rural older adults (Maiden & Peterson, 2002; Rost, Fortney, Zhang, Smith, & Smith, 1999; Thommasen, Lavanchy, Connelly,

Berkowitz, & Grzybowski, 2001). A previous study found that depressed rural individuals were approximately three times more likely to be admitted to a hospital for physical problems and for mental health problems than were depressed urban individuals (Rost, Zhang, Fortney, Smith, & Smith, 1998). That same study found that rural subjects reported significantly more suicide attempts during a one-year period. Research has found that rural residents with a history of depressive symptom are more likely to have a negative attitude about people who seek professional help for the disorder than are urban residents with the disorder (Rost, Smith, & Taylor, 1993). This study found that the more negative they were, the less likely they were to seek professional help for themselves. Barriers to the provision of, and the use of, effective outpatient specialty care must be surmounted in order for the rural health care system to provide proper care for depressed individuals. Rural individuals may be more likely to use primary care clinics because of their availability and relative closeness. Studies have shown that nonmedical factors, such as psychosocial issues, are an important reason for use of these clinics, and thus it is important that the medical providers in these clinics consider the psychosocial needs of this population (Mehl-Madrona, 1998). Yet in many cases the health care providers in these primary care clinics are overworked and dealing with emotional exhaustion and depression themselves (Thommasen, Lavanchy, Connelly, Berkowitz, & Grzybowski, 2001).

Of particular interest are the results of the analyses of use of antidepressants. Approximately 17% of the women in this sample had filled a prescription for at least one antidepressant in the 12-month follow-up period, with no significant difference between rural and urban women. Thus despite the fewer physician visits with codes for depression for rural women, they were as likely as urban women to fill prescriptions for antidepressants. As in the case of anxiolytics, there appears to have been a low number of physician visits involving diagnosis codes for depression (2.7% for rural and 3.5% for urban) in the one-year follow-up, especially when compared with the use of antidepressants during that same year. Again it is of some concern that the large number of both rural and urban women receiving prescriptions for antidepressants had probably been diagnosed in a previous year, and had no apparent follow-up diagnosis in our 12-month period. We again point out the dangers of continued issuance of prescriptions for psychotropic medications with no surveillance of the psychological disorder that prompted the prescription, particularly in the elderly. It may be that the physicians of these medicated elderly are monitoring their psychological disorders without coding a diagnosis. However, reimbursement from Medicare would require the diagnostic code, and medical practice guidelines should urge physicians to monitor and record their ICD-9 codes.

Although there appears to be no rural/urban difference in use of antidepressants in the 12-month follow-up period, examination of the two major types of antidepressants revealed that rural women were significantly more likely to be prescribed a TCA and less likely to be prescribed a SSRI, compared with urban women. Adjusting for demographic factors and number of mentally unhealthy days, the significant difference for SSRIs persisted, but the TCA difference only approached significance ($p = .09$). When looking at only those women who had filled a prescription for an antidepressant in the 12-month study period, the greater likelihood for rural women to have filled a prescription for a TCA, as compared with urban women, again approached significance ($p = .06$). Thus our findings suggest a greater use of TCAs by rural women who use antidepressants.

Despite these rural/urban differences, there appears to be a relatively high use of TCAs by both groups of women. Of those who filled an antidepressant prescription in the 12-month period, 36% of the rural women and 31% of the urban women had filled a prescription for a TCA. These findings are of concern because of the potential side effects of TCAs on the central nervous and cardiovascular systems, particularly in the elderly (Emslie & Judge, 2000). Use of TCAs has also been shown to lead to higher rates of discontinuation by patients (Donoghue, 2000); this is true for both the old tricyclics as well as the newer tricyclics (Barbui et al., 2000), and puts the patient at risk for a recurrence of depression (Isacsson, Boethius, Henriksson, Jones, & Bergman, 1999). Most of these researchers stress that SSRIs are the safer alternative for this older population. Although in our study, urban women were more likely to have filled a prescription for SSRIs than rural women, research has shown a trend of increasing prescription of SSRIs to rural older adults (Ganguli, Mulsant, Richards, Stoehr, & Mendelsohn, 1997).

The rural/urban differences in use of types of antidepressants cannot be explained by cost differentials, since this sample were all members of PACE, which covers all costs of a prescription after a small copayment. One explanation could be that some of the health care providers in rural areas may lack extensive knowledge concerning the dangers of TCAs for elderly, and the relatively safer alternatives of SSRIs. An important source of information about medications comes from the pharmaceutical representatives; perhaps they make fewer trips to the more remote rural primary health care centers.

Although we had found no overall rural/urban difference in the likelihood of a member of this sample to fill a prescription for any antidepressant, we looked more carefully at that segment of the sample who expressed the greatest problem with depressed mood: those who had reported 14 or more days of depressed mood in the past 30 days. Adjusting for demographic factors and number of depressed mood days, we found that rural women were less likely to have filled a prescription for an antidepressant in the 12-month period following their self-report of a high number of depressed days; however this finding only approached significance ($p = .067$). Again, this possible undertreatment of psychological problems of rural older women should be of great concern. Undertreatment of depression may place these women at greater risk for attempted suicide, hospitalization, and premature institutionalization (Neese, Abraham, & Buckwalter, 1999). Cost analyses have found that annual expenditures for outpatient depression treatment are lower for rural subjects compared with their urban counterparts, and that for every dollar invested in depression treatment, there was a $2.61 decrease in the cost of treating physical problems in depressed rural residents (Rost et al., 1999). The human suffering associated with undertreatment of depression is harder to quantify but even more salient.

There are several limitations to this study. Compared with the general U.S. elderly population, PACE enrollees include a smaller proportion of minorities and married individuals. PACE enrollees are also older and have a lower annual income. Therefore, caution should be taken when generalizing these results. As with any study utilizing claims data, care must also be taken in making inferences about physician prescribing behavior based solely on pharmacy claims. For example, it is possible that some women who were prescribed an antidepressant or an anxiolytic agent did not fill the prescription. Also, we had no data on use of alternative therapy to deal with depressed mood or anxiety.

Results of this study indicate possible underutilization of antide-pressants among rural women, as well as possible overuse of anxio-lytics. Future research is needed to examine the reasons for these prescription drug use patterns, as well as the reasons for the lower rate of physician visits with codes for depression among rural women compared with urban women, despite similar self-reports of number of depressed mood days. It is of utmost importance that older rural women receive high quality medical care from providers who are trained in mental health assessment and treatment.

REFERENCES

Barbui, C., Hotopf, M., Freemantle, N., Boynton, J., Churchill, R., Eccles, M. P., et al. (2000). Selective serotonin reuptake inhibitors versus tricyclic and heterocyclic antidepressants: comparison of drug adherence. *Cochrane Database System Review, 4*, CD002791.

Borawski, E., Wu, G., & Jia, H. (1998). Self-reported frequent mental distress among adults-United States, 1993–1996. *Morbidity and Mortality Weekly Report, 47*(16), 325–331.

Craig, D., Passmore, A. P., Fullerton, K. J., Beringer, T. R., Gilmore, D. H., Crawford, V., et al. (2003). Factors influencing prescription of CNS medications in different elderly populations. *Pharmacoepidemiological and Drug Safety, 5*, 383–387.

Donoghue, J. (2000). Antidepressant use patterns in clinical practices: Comparisons among tricyclic antidepressants and selective serotonin reuptake inhibitors. *Acta Psychiatry Scandinavian Supplement, 403*, 57–61.

Diagnostic and Statistical Manual of Mental Disorders (DSM-IV, 4th ed.) (1994). Washington, DC: American Psychiatric Association.

Durch, J. S., Bailey, L. A., & Stoto, M. A. (Eds.). (1997). *Improving Health in the Community: A Role for Performance Monitoring.* Washington, DC: The National Academy Press.

Emslie, G., & Judge, R. (2000). Tricyclic antidepressants and selective serotonin reuptake inhibitors: Use during pregnancy, in children/adolescents and in the elderly. *Acta Psychiatry Scandinavian Supplement, 403*, 26–34.

Esposito, L. (1994). Home health case management: Rural caregiving. *Home Healthcare Nurse, 12*(3), 38–43.

Fortney, J., Rost, K., Zhang, M., & Warren, J. (1999). The impact of geographic accessibility on the intensity and quality of depression treatment. *Medical Care, 37*(9), 884–893.

Fox, J. C., Blank, M., Berman, J., & Rovnyak, V. (1999). Mental disorders and help seeking in a rural impoverished population. *International Journal of Psychiatry Medicine, 29*, 181–195.

Fried, L., & Wallace, R. (1992). The complexity of chronic illness in the elderly: From clinic to community. In R. Wallace & R. Woolson (Eds.), *The epidemiologic study of the elderly.* New York: Oxford University Press.

Gale, B. J. (1993). Psychosocial health needs of older women: Urban versus rural comparisons. *Archives of Psychiatric Nursing, 7*(2), 99–105.

Ganguli, M., Mulsant, B., Richards, S., Stoehr, G., & Mendelsohn, A. (1997). Antidepressant use over time in a rural older adult population: The MoVIES Project. *Journal of the American Geriatric Society, 45*(12), 1501–1503.

Horsley, S., Barrow, S., Gent, N., & Astbury, J. (1998). Informal care and psychiatric morbidity. *Journal of Public Health Medicine, 20*(2), 180–185.

Isacsson, G., Boethius, G., Henriksson, S., Jones, J. K., & Bergman, U. (1999). Selective serotonin reuptake inhibitors have broadened the utilization of antidepressant treatment in accordance with recommendations: Findings from a Swedish prescription database. *Journal of Affective Disorders, 53*(1), 15–22.

Maiden, R. J., & Peterson, S. A. (2002). Use of mental health services by the rural aged: Longitudinal study. *Journal of Geriatric Psychiatry and Neurology, 15*(1), 1–6.

Mehl-Madrona, L. E. (1998). Frequent users of rural primary care: Comparisons with randomly selected users. *Journal of the American Board of Family Practice, 11*(2), 105–115.

Mort, J. R., & Aparasu, R. R. (2000). Prescribing potentially inappropriate psychotropic medications to the ambulatory elderly. *Archives of Internal Medicine, 160*(18), 2825–2831.

Mort, J. R., Gaspar, P. M., Juffer, D. I., & Kovarna, M. B. (1996). Comparison of psychotropic agent use among rural elderly caregivers and noncaregivers. *Annals of Pharmacotherapy, 30*(6), 583–585.

Neese, J. B., Abraham, I. L., & Buckwalter, K. C. (1999). Utilization of mental health services among rural elderly. *Archives of Psychiatric Nursing, 13*, 30–40.

Reed, D. B., & Claunch, D. T. (2002). Behind the scenes: Spousal coping following permanently disabling injury of farmers. *Issues in Mental Health Nursing, 23*(3), 231–248.

Revicki, D. A., & Mitchell, J. P. (1990). Strain, social support, and mental health in rural elderly individuals. *Journal of Gerontology, 45*, S267–S274.

Rost, K., Fortney, J., Zhang, M., Smith, J., & Smith, G. R., Jr. (1999). Treatment of depression in rural Arkansas: Policy implications for improving care. *Journal of Rural Health, 15*(3), 308–315.

Rost, K., Smith, G. R., & Taylor, J. L. (1993). Rural-urban differences in stigma and the use of care for depressive disorders. *Journal of Rural Health, 9*(1), 57–62.

Rost, K., Zhang, M., Fortney, J., Smith, J., & Smith G. R., Jr. (1998). Rural-urban differences in depression treatment and suicidality. *Medical Care, 36*(7), 1098–1107.

Rural Policy Research Institute (1999). Rural-Urban Continuum Codes: Definitions from the Economic Research Service, USDA. Available at http://www.rupri.org/resources/context/ers-ruc.html

Russell, D. W., Cutrona, C. E., de la Mora, A., & Wallace, R. B. (1997). Loneliness and nursing home admission among rural older adults. *Psychology and Aging, 12*(4), 574–589.

Sanford, J. T., & Townsend-Rocchiccioli, J. (2004). The perceived health of rural caregivers. *Geriatric Nursing, 25*(3), 145–148.

Thommasen, H. V., Lavanchy, M., Connelly, I., Berkowitz, J., & Grzybowski, S. (2001). Mental health, job satisfaction, and intention to relocate. Opinions of physicians in rural British Columbia. *Canadian Family Physician, 47*, 737–744.

Watts, P. R., Dinger, M. K., Baldwin, K. A., Sisk, R. J., Brockschmidt, B. A., & McCubbin, J. E. (1999). Accessibility and perceived value of health services in five western Illinois rural communities. *Journal of Community Health, 24*(2), 147–157.

Chapter 4

Obesity in Rural Women: Emerging Risk Factors and Hypotheses

Christine M. Olson and Caron F. Bove

OVERVIEW

This chapter begins with an introduction to the topic of obesity and then discusses two research papers that were presented at the 2002 Rural Women's Health Conference in Washington, DC. Each study examines possible factors involved in the development of obesity in rural women. The first study addresses the association between one specific factor, food insecurity, and obesity. We provide an overview of the literature on this relatively new topic and then present the methods and results of a secondary analysis of data from an NIH-funded project (HD 29549) on rural women's weight gain. The second study is an in-depth qualitative study designed to identify a range of possible factors contributing to the development of obesity in a sample of rural low-income women from upstate New York. This study's methods and results, the latter in the form of emergent themes and hypotheses, are presented. This chapter concludes with a discussion of both of the studies presented in this chapter.

INTRODUCTION

Obesity is a highly prevalent and growing nutrition problem among women in the United States. Obesity is associated with adverse health outcomes, including increased risk for hypertension, Type 2 diabetes mellitus, cardiovascular disease, osteoarthritis, gallbladder disease, and some cancers (Pi-Sunyer, 1993), as well as social stigmatization (Sobal, 1999). In 1999 and 2000, 33.4% of adult women age 20 years and older were obese with a body mass index (BMI) of 30 or greater, according to the National Health and Nutrition Examination Survey (NHANES; Flegal, Carroll, Ogden, & Johnson, 2002). (BMI is an indicator of percentage of body fat and is expressed as body weight in kilograms [kg] divided by the square of height in meters [m], or kg/m^2.) Obesity varied by age with women 50 to 70 years having the highest prevalence. Obesity varied more dramatically by racial/ethnic group with non-Hispanic Whites showing a prevalence of 30.1%, non-Hispanic Blacks 49.7%, and Mexican Americans 39.7%. The prevalence of obesity among women ages 20 to 74 years increased from 25.9% in 1988–1994 to 34.0% in 1999–2000, representing a dramatic increase from 1976–1980 when the prevalence was 17.0%.

The racial/ethnic differences cited above very likely illustrate the well-known differences in obesity across socioeconomic strata. In 2000, using self-reported weights from the Behavioral Risk Factor Surveillance Survey (BRFSS), Mokdad and colleagues (2001) found nearly a twofold difference in the prevalence of obesity by educational level, an indicator of socioeconomic status. Twenty-six percent of adults with less than a high school education were obese, compared with 15% of those with a college degree or higher education.

Until fairly recently, little research has been done on geographic area of residence as a potential risk factor for obesity. Using data from NHANES II, Sobal, Troiano, and Frongillo (1996) found rural White women were on average about 5 pounds heavier than their urban counterparts. Obesity varied more by urbanization for women than it did for men according to data from the National Health Interview Survey (Eberhardt et al., 2001; McIntosh & Sobal, 2004). In 1997–1998, women in the fringe counties of large metro areas had the lowest age-adjusted prevalence of obesity (16%), whereas women in the most rural counties had the highest prevalence (23%). Interestingly, the county type with the highest prevalence of obesity varied by area of the United States. The pattern above was present in the Northeast and South; in the Midwest and the West, however, women in central counties with large metropolitan areas had the highest rates of obesity (25% and 18% respectively).

The socioeconomic gradient in obesity seen in women nationally is also prominent in rural areas. In a survey of the entire population of a rural county in upstate New York, Pearson and Lewis (1998) found a strong inverse relationship between educational level and obesity (defined as a BMI of 27.3 or greater) in all age groups of women from 17 to 65 years. This was most evident in women 30 to 49 years, among whom the prevalence of obesity was 37% for those with less than high school education and 16% for those who were college graduates. It is hypothesized that the lower socioeconomic status of rural people may be at least part of the explanation for the higher rates of obesity seen in rural areas. In support of this hypothesis, Sobal and colleagues (1996) found that the 5-pound weight difference between rural and urban White women disappeared when demographic and behavioral variables were considered in the regression analysis.

The dramatic increase in obesity seen in recent years in national samples also appears to be present in rural areas. In a study of the change in weight from 1992 to 1997 in adults residing in a rural Wisconsin county, Rothacker and Blackburn (2000) found that women gained an average of 7.3 kg and the prevalence of overweight and obesity increased by 11% and 13%, respectively. The incidence, or new cases, of overweight and obesity was particularly dramatic. Only 48% of the women who were normal weight in 1992 remained so in 1997, with 45% becoming overweight and 8% becoming obese. The youngest age group of women (age 20 to 30 years) showed the greatest five-year increase in body weight (11.0 kg). These researchers concluded that "research is needed to identify specific causal factors of the age-related weight gain" (Rothacker & Blackburn, 2000).

STUDY 1: THE PARADOX OF FOOD INSECURITY AND OBESITY

We recently undertook a study to confirm our previous research on food insecurity as a contributor to the higher prevalence of obesity in lower income women. In this study we used an expert panel's definition of food insecurity: "Food insecurity exists whenever the availability of nutritionally adequate and safe food or the ability to acquire acceptable foods in socially acceptable ways is limited or uncertain" (Anderson, 1990). Hunger, a narrower and more severe form of deprivation, was defined as "the painful or uneasy sensation caused by a lack of food" (Anderson, 1990).

Background

Food insecurity and hunger have been assessed annually since 1995 in nationally representative samples of the U.S. population as part of the Current Population Survey. In 2001, the most recent year for which national data are available, 10.7% of U.S. households (11.5 million households) were food insecure and 3.3% (3.5 million households) were food insecure with hunger (Nord, Andrews, & Carlson, 2002).

Food insecurity in the U.S. varies substantially by household characteristics. In 2001, households with incomes below the federal poverty line had a prevalence of food insecurity that was 36.5%, over three times the national average (Nord, Andrews, & Carlson, 2002). Black and Hispanic households had prevalences of 21.3% and 21.8%, respectively. The prevalence of food insecurity also varies geographically across the U.S. In 2001, central city and nonmetropolitan households had food insecurity prevalences of 13.9% and 11.5%, respectively, compared with 8.3% in metropolitan households outside central cities.

In a 1993 random sample survey in a rural county in upstate New York, Olson (1999) showed that BMI was significantly higher ($p < 0.05$) for women in food-insecure households compared with women in food-secure households (28.2 vs. 25.6). In addition, 37% of the women in the food insecure households had BMIs greater than 29 and were designated as obese, compared with 26% of women in food-secure households. Food insecurity was still positively related to BMI even when we controlled for the women's height, income level, educational level, single-parent status, and employment status (Frongillo, Olson, Rauschenbach, & Kendall, 1997).

Townsend, Peerson, Love, Achterberg, and Murphy (2001) recently replicated this finding in women, using nationally representative data. The prevalence of overweight (BMI > 27.3) increased as food insecurity became more severe, from 34% for those who were food secure, to 41% for those who were mildly food insecure, and to 52% for those who were moderately food insecure.

One of the major remaining research questions concerns the mechanisms by which food insecurity leads to obesity in women. Radimer, Olson, Greene, Campbell, and Habicht's (1992) early qualitative research on food insecurity documented that mothers go without food, particularly at times when food and money for food are limited, to ensure that their children have something to eat. The eating pattern literature supports the idea that food deprivation could result in overeating. Polivy (1996) found that food restriction and deprivation, whether voluntary or involuntary, result in a variety of cognitive, emotional and behavioral changes such as preoccupation with food and eating.

In the 1993 study, Kendall, Olson and Frongillo (1996) found a positive linear association between the severity of food insecurity and a binge-like pattern of eating. When an eating pattern score was added to a logistic regression model predicting obesity that included food-insecurity variables and other covariates, it was significant (p = .02) and the parameter estimate for food security decreased slightly (Frongillo, Olson, Rauschenback, & Kendall, 1997).

The new study reported here aims to confirm the relationship of food insecurity to obesity and also to determine whether a disordered pattern of eating is related to food insecurity and to obesity in a sample of rural women.

Methods

To address these research objectives, we undertook a secondary analysis of data from a prospective cohort study of 622 healthy adult (≥ 18 years) women who were followed from early pregnancy until two years postpartum.[1] The sample was recruited from the population of women who registered for obstetrical care over a two-year period in a hospital and primary care clinic system serving a rural, 10-county area of upstate New York. The population and sample were primarily White (96%) and socioeconomically diverse.

Three methods of data collection were employed. The women were mailed questionnaires at each of four time periods: first or second trimester of pregnancy, six months postpartum, and one and two years postpartum. Shortly after delivery, the women's obstetrical records were audited and the data entered directly into a computer. In addition, body weight and height were measured following study protocols (empty bladder, no shoes, and street clothing) by health care providers at antenatal visits and one and two years postpartum.

The data for this study come from the two-year postpartum time point. The food insecurity variable and the disordered eating pattern variables were created from questions on the mailed two-year-postpartum questionnaire. The three items measuring the least severe level of food insecurity from the U.S. Department of Agriculture's U.S. Household Food Security Survey Module were used to measure food insecurity. A positive response to any one of the items indicated the household was food insecure (Bickel, Nord, Price, Hamilton, & Cook, 2000). Four items from a scale developed by Agras (1987) were used as the measure for a disordered pattern of eating. An example of an item from this scale is "Do you ever eat large quantities of food deliberately out of the sight of other people? Yes or No." The medical record provided the information on women's sociodemographic characteristics. Data were analyzed using logistic regression analysis, first one predictor variable at a time (bivariate) and then those with a p-value of < .10 were included in a multivariate model. Known confounding variables—being a single parent, low income (≤ 185% of the Federal poverty line), educational level, age, and number of servings of fruits and vegetables eaten each day (as an indicator of dietary quality)—were included in the regression models.

Results

Both weight and food insecurity data were available for 411 women. In this sample, 24.6% were obese (BMI > 29), 20.4% lived in food-insecure households, and 42.1% indicated a disordered pattern of eating. Table 4.1 shows the results from both the bivariate and multivariate logistic regression analyses. Food insecurity and disordered eating were both positively and independently associated with obesity. In the multivariate analysis, women who lived in food-insecure households were almost twice as likely to be obese than

TABLE 4.1   The Association of Food Insecurity and Other Factors With Risk of Obesity (BMI > 29) in Rural Women

Factor	Bivariate Analysis		Multivariate Analysis	
	Odds Ratio	p Value	Odds Ratio	p Value
Food Insecurity	2.47	< .001	1.73	.05
Disordered Eating	3.19	< .001	2.72	< .001
Single Parent	1.83	.09	–[a]	–
Low Income[b]	1.93	.003	–	–
Educational Level[c]	0.35	< .001	0.47	.01
No. Fruits & Vegetables[c]	0.58	.03	–	–
Age[c]	0.52	.004	0.66	.10

[a]Variable not included in the multivariate model.
[b]"Low income" is defined as "a household income of less than 185% of the Federal poverty line.
[c]These variables are included in the models as continuous variables.

women who lived in food-secure households. Women who had a disordered or more binge-like pattern of eating were almost three times more likely to be obese. Two other variables remained in the multivariate model: education and age. Higher educational level was protective against obesity, as was older age. Further analysis showed that food insecurity was also significantly associated with disordered eating (p < .001). Sixty-eight percent of the food-secure women had no indication of a disordered pattern of eating, but only 39% of the food-insecure women had no indication of disordered eating.

STUDY 2: POTENTIAL RISK FACTORS FOR OBESITY IN RURAL LOW-INCOME WOMEN

Background

The obesity research presented thus far has used quantitative survey methods, which, although useful for assessing the prevalence of obesity in specific populations, do not provide insights into the social, situational, and cultural contexts of obesity. We undertook this next study, therefore, to develop an understanding of body weight as it is experienced by a group of women at risk for overweight and obesity. Using qualitative research methods, which are useful in health research for understanding complex issues that are poorly understood by closed-ended questions (Giacomini & Cook, 2000), we sought to understand rural low-income women's everyday experiences related to body weight and to identify structural barriers to weight maintenance that are unique to rural locales.

Methods

We collected the data for this investigation in upstate New York as part of a longitudinal multistate research project entitled "Rural Low-Income Families: Tracking Their Well-Being and Functioning in the Context of Welfare Reform" (Rural Families Speak, 2002).[2] In the multistate project, more than 400 rural low-income families from 15 states across the U.S. are being followed to analyze interrelationships among welfare policy, community programs and supports, individual and family circumstances, and overall family wellbeing. Our research aims for the New York State data also include the elucidation of factors contributing to obesity in rural low-income women.

We recruited our sample of 30 women and their families from rural communities in two nonmetropolitan counties in upstate New York. One county is completely rural, with no village of more than 2,500 people. The other county has one small city with a population of about 19,000; we recruited participants from the rural communities outside of this urban area.

Data collection occurred in 3 waves over a three-year period. In-depth, personal interviews used both closed- and open-ended questions focused on several specific topics: living in the community, family of origin, employment, child care, transportation, housing, income and making ends meet, food security, health, parenting, and social support. In New York State we collected supplementary data on the mother in each participating household: each woman's measured body weight; her self-reported height; her perceptions of her weight; and information about her daily activities and eating patterns (including questions that focus on disordered eating [Agras, 1987] and stress-related dietary changes). Interviews lasting $1^1/2$ to 3 hours were audiotaped, transcribed verbatim, and verified against the audiotapes. To date the first and second waves of data have been collected, and they provide the data for this analysis. All participating family members were assigned pseudonyms to maintain their anonymity.

Qualitative data are being analyzed using the constant comparative method (Glaser & Strauss, 1967; Strauss & Corbin, 1990). Data collection and analysis occurred simultaneously, with analyses of Wave 1 and Wave 2 interviews informing the collection and analysis of Wave 3 data. Our analysis uses both case-based and concept-based approaches (Miles & Huberman, 1994). Analysis is an iterative process employing both hypothesis generation and hypothesis testing, and our conceptual framework is evolving to eventually include all three waves of data.

Results

Characteristics of the Women

At the time of first interviews, the mothers residing in the 30 New York households were 19 to 48 years old, and most were in their 20s or 30s. Eighty percent had attained a high school diploma, and nearly one-half of all women had received some education beyond high school, typically technical training. Only one woman had completed a four-year college degree. Twenty-five women resided with a male partner, and of these, 16 were married to the partner. One to seven children resided in these households. Twenty-seven (90%) of the women described themselves as White, one as Black, and two as multiracial.

Women's BMIs were calculated and categorized according to recent national guidelines (National Heart, Lung, and Blood Institute [NHLBI] Obesity Task Force, 1998). One-third of women were obese (BMI ≥ 30.0), 23% were overweight (BMI 25.0–29.9), 37% were normal weight (BMI 18.5–24.9), and 7% were underweight (BMI < 18.5).

Emergent Themes

Although we had been interested from the outset in studying body weight in rural women, we had focused initially on women's eating habits (in terms of food insecurity, disordered eating, and stress-induced eating) rather than consider both dietary and physical activity behaviors. What emerged from our preliminary analysis of the women's interviews, however, was variation in body weight that seemed to relate to the coexistence of several factors that underlay their levels of physical activity: the women's place of residence, their transportation difficulties, their employment, and their physical and mental health. Thus, consideration of women's physical activity patterns, in addition to their eating behaviors, was vital for understanding differences in these women's weights. In addition, while specific characteristics appeared to differentiate normal-weight women from obese, the overweight women shared some characteristics with obese women, but others with normal-weight women. Thus this presentation primarily contrasts obese with normal-weight women, discussing overweight women where it seems most appropriate.

Patterns Common to Obese Women

With one exception, obese and overweight women perceived themselves as overweight and heavier than they desired. That they were disappointed in their weight was clear from their comments, for example, "I don't like to be fat! I want to lose weight!" The obese women in particular were "not happy with it," typically desiring weight loss "for health reasons." All had been told by a health care professional that they were overweight. Three obese women were trying to lose weight at the time of their Wave 2 interviews.

Disordered eating appeared to be common to obese and overweight women. Some women said they tended to eat a lot of food quickly if they skipped a meal; others indicated that they ate only one meal a day, at which time they usually "pig out." Some said that they binged: "Yes, there's times I've done that. . . . Probably 'cause I go days without eating and then I'll make up for it." Eliza, a 34-year-old mother of eight, perceived her eating pattern as unusual in "how much I eat. I eat more when I'm depressed. Yeah, when I'm depressed I just find myself eating just to be eating." Two women, one obese and one overweight, were notable for perceiving not only that they ate far less than other people but also that they could go for days, even weeks, without eating, for example:

> It's very abnormal. Once a day, IF I feel like it. 'Cause I don't like food. I can go two, three days before I get hungry enough where

I need somethin'. As long as I have my coffee and my water I'm happy.—Steph

'Cause there's times I don't [eat], I can go weeks without eatin'. I can go weeks without eatin'. I won't even think of food.—Lee

Transportation issues and physical activity opportunities and behaviors were closely intertwined. A considerable proportion of women in our sample, but obese women in particular, periodically found themselves without reliable transportation. These rural communities have little public transportation, forcing families to depend on their own vehicles or on the kindness of others for transportation. Whereas a mother might request assistance from extended family, friends, or neighbors to transport a sick child to a hospital in an emergency, she would be less inclined to ask for help on a daily basis. Transportation problems meant that some women had difficulty leaving their homes, particularly to go places as a family unit, which limited women's prospects for physical activity. One obese woman was homebound in a remote part of the county during the winter months when her husband used their only reliable vehicle for commuting to work. Other women's activities were limited not only by their partner's using the household's sole vehicle for commuting to work, but also by their vehicles—usually pick-up trucks— being too small to transport the women and their children simultaneously.

In addition to the lack of transportation, other structural factors constrained women's physical activity. Although these families resided in rural communities, they were not involved in intense manual labor such as farming. Their homes typically were small mobile homes or apartments, usually on one level, often without stairs. Homes were located along highways where there were no sidewalks and few streetlights, despite the frequent passing of vehicles. Walking was difficult in this setting, especially with young children and strollers.

Obese women were less likely to be employed than either overweight or normal-weight women, with unemployment contributing to obese women's lower levels of physical activity as well as to their isolation at home. For some obese women employment was not possible on account of chronic physical health problems:

There's a lot of pain. It's hard for me to get around. If I'm on my feet too much I have to use either a cane or a walker 'cause my legs will give out on me. If I go to the grocery store, I can't take too much of the walk. I have to use a wheelchair.—Zola

For other obese women, mental health problems underlay their unemployment:

I had a nervous breakdown . . . and haven't been able to get back to work since. I worked for three months and left the job on the verge of another nervous breakdown . . . I have depression. Um, anxiety and panic disorder. Agoraphobia. That's fear of public places or going outside.—Bevin

Bevin's "nervous breakdown" was the culmination of her learning of her children's sexual abuse at the hands of their father, along with her family's plummet from its "upper-middle-class rather snobby background" to "facing possibly homelessness" and "financial debt that I never, never could have anticipated" when her marriage dissolved. Her depression impeded her ability to be employed, further compromising her children's economic security and enhancing her sense of despair. Interwoven with her sense of futility were her feelings about her obesity ("It's horrible!") that further inhibited her from stepping outside her home, held her back in seeking employment, and perhaps further hindered her recovery from depression.

It [weight] affects all areas, you know! Any time we leave this house, you know, I'm aware of every pound and how I look and how I measure up depending on where we're going. . . . Logically I can say it shouldn't be this way, but you know, for me, yeah, it's always there. So, it does, it holds me back from doing things in all areas that I'd like to do.—Bevin

Musculoskeletal difficulties limiting employment also restricted some obese and overweight women's domestic and parenting activities, as one obese woman's husband explained:

I guess it affects us with a lot of the health problems she has in the wintertime because we don't, she can't get out a lot. So there's a lot of things that we can't do out there that we need to do. . . . It limits what you can, how much you can tolerate as far as doin' housework and doin' stuff with your kids.

Patterns Common to Normal-Weight Women

Most normal-weight women perceived their weight as "all right" or "fine" and said little about weight in general. Those who wanted to lose weight tended to have been pregnant within the previous year and desired to return to their prepregnancy weight but were "not real worried" about doing so.

Disordered eating appeared to be uncommon among normal-weight women. Affirmative responses to the disordered eating questions sounded typical of women leading busy lives, for example, that a woman would occasionally lack the time to eat a meal or that she would eat quickly because she was busy. Lorilei said, "I eat fast just because . . . I eat when the kids are sleepin' or busy. And at work we don't have time to sit there and, you know, sit down and eat a decent meal."

Whereas transportation constraints and limitations in physical activity were prominent themes in the interviews with obese women, this was not the case in interviews with normal-weight women. What emerged from normal-weight women's narratives instead was the importance of walking in these women's lives and/or the facility with which they were able to walk given their residing in the population centers of their communities. In these populated areas with sidewalks and streetlights, women walked to commute to their places of employment ("I walk to work all the time"), to run errands ("If I need anything I'm within walking distance"), to socialize with friends and relatives, and for relaxation and stress relief. Describing how she spent time with friends, one woman said:

> Go to baseball games. And then we go four-wheeling. We walk. Some of my other friends, we just walk . . . I'll call my best friend up and I'll say, "Hey, let's go for a walk or something." And we'll walk down to the pier, back up around by A-Plus [a convenience store] and across the street and back down, you know.—Emeline

Emeline also spoke of walking as a means to unwind after work:

> I do go for a couple occasional walks after I get done with work . . . when I get stressed out from work I like to go for a walk because it relaxes a person, and then I come home and I'm fine.

Thus for women living in the more populated, commercial regions of their rural communities, being without a vehicle did not mean that they would be homebound. They had an alternative —walking.

Tracy, a normal-weight woman who moved from a rural community to a more urban setting during her participation in our project, exemplified this rural-urban difference. At the time of her first interview, Tracy was confined with her husband and two young children to a small, dilapidated mobile home in a remote part of the county where even a leisurely walk up the road was hindered by fast-moving traffic.

> *Tracy:* You get lonely, you don't got no friends, you can't go anywhere. And it's like . . . if I could just go out on a sidewalk and just take a decent walk, without no one bothering you, then that's, I like that.
>
> *Husband:* Yeah, but you can't do that here. Trucks go by here 80 miles per hour.
>
> *Tracy:* Oh, people drive through! You get Mac trucks over here, because of the farming. I mean they go through here 60, 70 miles an hour. And, that's even cars. I mean, my grandmother's dog just got hit, by his leg, 'cause a car didn't stop and slow down.

Concerns about rabid animals had further hampered Tracy's outdoor activities, contributing to her loneliness and depression. When asked how she liked her rural neighborhood as a place to live, Tracy replied:

> I don't like it, I guess you could say. I don't think it's safe. 'Cause, we are in the country, and most animals around here, they pretty much respect our privacy and don't come down, but occasionally when they do it's, you know, you just can't walk outside. Like this past summer we had a bobcat that's running around. . . . So you can't just go outside and take a walk with your kids if you choose to. . . . If anything's rabid, then you better start running as fast as you can. That's pretty hard with two kids.

By the time of her second interview, Tracy and her family had moved to the small city within their county. Although Tracy complained about her new neighborhood, she nonetheless enjoyed living within walking distance of shops, which she could visit for buying essentials or for leisure-time activity: "I'm close to Ames. It's about a 10-minute walk to Ames, which is nice. Which has Kinney Drugs,

Ames. It's nice to go and look." The family's move to the county seat not only enabled Tracy to better manage without a vehicle, but she perceived that it had also facilitated her postpartum weight loss: "It's like, 'How can I get there? I've got two feet. I know how to use them. It ain't gonna hurt me.' I walk. Actually, I've lost a lot of my [postpartum] weight that way."

Normal-weight women in general did not experience the constraints that confined some obese women to their homes. Normal-weight women tended not to be limited in their physical activities, including their ability to be employed, by musculoskeletal, respiratory, and mental health problems to the same degree as obese women. Normal-weight women were employed in a variety of jobs, including waitress, postal worker, convenience store clerk, nurses' aide, school cafeteria worker, and daycare provider. Normal-weight women residing in population centers were physically able to run errands, walk to work, and be active outside their homes even in the absence of an automobile.

DISCUSSION

Body weight in rural low-income women is a complex, multifaceted phenomenon. Interwoven into the fabric of overweight and obesity is food insecurity occurring within the context of rural isolation, unemployment, limited opportunities for household and leisure-time physical activities, chronic physical and mental health problems, and distorted eating patterns. The quantitative analysis in Study 1 confirmed that food insecurity was a rural area. In addition, Study 1 demonstrates that disordered eating is related to food insecurity and is also independently related to obesity. These findings suggest that, although it may seem counterintuitive, rural families need certain and consistent access to sufficient nutritious food, including maximum participation in the Federal Food and Nutrition Assistance Programs and food and nutrition education, as protection against obesity because food insecurity increases a woman's risk of being obese.

Study 1 has certain limitations. All of the research reported to date comes from cross-sectional studies, with data for the two major constructs (obesity and food insecurity) collected at the same point in time. Thus, we are constrained in specifying the direction of causality between the two constructs. Longitudinal data could inform the direction of causality by facilitating analysis that considers the temporal sequence of the two constructs. For example, is food insecurity at Time 1 related to the risk of becoming overweight at Time 2 and to major weight gain between the two time points? This research is needed before definitive conclusions can be drawn about relationships between food insecurity and obesity.

The qualitative approach of Study 2 provides contextual depth to our understanding of body weight in rural economically disadvantaged women. Rural low-income mothers residing outside of village centers are perhaps at particular risk for obesity due to transportation and other problems that confine women to their homes and contribute to sedentary lifestyles. That the transportation challenges of rural areas act as barriers to physical activity is consistent with the structural barriers hypothesized to exist in rural areas by other authors (Tai-Seale & Chandler, 2003). The rural-urban difference in body weight and physical activity level that is emerging from this qualitative investigation finds support in Pearson and Lewis's study (1998) of another rural, upstate New York county in which lower obesity rates were found among residents of a small city than among the more rural population, regardless of educational attainment. Findings from our current as well as our earlier qualitative research (Devine, Bove, & Olson, 2000) suggest: a) physical activity, like walking, that can be incorporated into the activities of daily living is the most accessible and thus the most likely form of physical activity to be performed by women with young children, especially by women of limited economic means; b) in rural communities walking is most easily performed by women residing in populated areas where sidewalks, streetlights, and relatively slow-moving traffic as well as nearby, closely spaced destinations, i.e., schools, shops, libraries, healthcare and other services, and neighbors, allow it to be integrated most smoothly into women's domestic and parenting activities; and c) walking appears to play an important role in women's weight management. Other researchers (e.g., Rothacker & Blackburn, 2000) have suggested that the large distances from homes to stores and neighbors force rural residents to rely on automobiles for travel, thereby contributing to sedentary lifestyles. Our study reveals that the absence of functioning, adequately sized automobiles in some low-income rural households enforces sedentary life-styles even further.

The findings of Study 2 represent preliminary work only. Additional data collection and analysis to further elucidate the phenomenon of obesity in this population is on-going and will consider interrelationships among body weight, food insecurity, disordered eating, stress-induced eating behaviors, and cigarette smoking.

NOTES

1. Support for the secondary data analysis was provided by a Small Grant from the University of California at Davis provided by the Economic Research Service, Food & Economic Division of the U.S. Department of Agriculture (Grant 43–3AEM–1–80038).
2. Support for this research was provided by the Agricultural Experiment Stations and Cooperative Extension in the cooperating states (see below), and Ohio University, Maryland Department of Human Resources, American Association of Family and Consumer Sciences, and U.S. Department of Agriculture (NRICGP2000–0159, NRICGP2001–35401–10215, NRICGP2002–35401–11591). Cooperating states: California, Colorado, Indiana, Kentucky, Louisiana, Maryland, Massachusetts, Michigan, Minnesota, Nebraska, New Hampshire, New York (Cornell University Project NYC–399401), Ohio, Oregon, and Wyoming.

REFERENCES

Agras, W. S. (1987). *Eating disorders: Management of obesity, bulimia, and anorexia nervosa*. New York: Pergamon Press.

Anderson, S. A. (Ed.). (1990). Core indicators of nutritional status for difficult-to-sample populations. *Journal of Nutrition, 120,* 1559–1600.

Bickel, G., Nord, M., Price, C., Hamilton, W., & Cook, J. (2000). *Guide to measuring household food security*. Alexandria, VA: U.S. Department of Agriculture, Food and Nutrition Service.

Devine, C. M., Bove, C. F., & Olson, C. M. (2000). Continuity and change in women's weight orientations and lifestyle practices through pregnancy and the postpartum period: The influence of life course trajectories and transitional events. *Social Science & Medicine, 50,* 567–582.

Eberhardt, M. S., Ingram, D. D., Makuc, D. M., Pamuk, E. R., Freid, V. M., Harper, S. B., et al. (2001). *Urban and rural health chartbook: Health, United States, 2001*. Hyattsville, MD: National Center for Health Statistics.

Flegal, K. A., Carroll, M. D., Ogden, C. L., & Johnson, C. L. (2002). Prevalence and trends in obesity among U.S. adults, 1999–2000. *Journal of the American Medical Association, 288,* 1723–1727.

Frongillo, E. A., Jr., Olson, C. M., Rauschenbach, B. S., & Kendall, A. (1997). *Nutritional consequences of food insecurity in a rural New York State county* (Discussion Paper No. 1120–97). Institute for Research on Poverty, University of Wisconsin-Madison, Madison, WI.

Giacomini, M. K., & Cook, D. J. (2000). Users' guides to the medical literature: XXIII. Qualitative research in health care A: Are the results of the study valid? *Journal of the American Medical Association, 284*(3), 357–362.

Glaser, B., & Strauss, A. (1967). *The discovery of grounded theory: Strategies for qualitative research.* Chicago: Aldine.

Kendall, A., Olson, C. M., & Frongillo, E. A., Jr. (1996). Relationship of hunger and food insecurity to food availability and consumption. *Journal of the American Dietetic Association, 96,* 1019–1024.

McIntosh, W. A., & Sobal, J. (2004). Rural eating, diet, nutrition, and body weight. In N. Glasgow, L. W. Morton, & N. E. Johnson (Eds.), *Critical issues in rural health.* Ames, IA: Blackwell.

Miles, M. B., & Huberman, A. M. (1994). *Qualitative data analysis: An expanded sourcebook.* Thousand Oaks, CA: Sage.

Mokdad, A. H., Bowman, B. A., Ford, E. S., Vinicor, F., Marks, J. S., & Koplan, J. P. (2001). The continuing epidemics of obesity and diabetes in the United States. *Journal of the American Medical Association, 286,* 1195–1200.

National Heart, Lung, and Blood Institute Obesity Task Force (1998). Clinical guidelines on the identification, evaluation, and treatment of overweight and obesity in adults: The evidence report. *Obesity Research, 6*(Suppl. 2), 51S–209S.

Nord, M., Andrews, M., & Carlson, S. (2002). *Household food security in the United States, 2001* (FANRR-29). Alexandria, VA: Food and Rural Economics Division, Economic Research Service, U.S. Department of Agriculture.

Olson, C. M. (1999). Nutrition and health outcomes associated with food insecurity and hunger. *Journal of Nutrition, 129,* 521S–524S.

Pearson, T. A., & Lewis, C. (1998). Rural epidemiology: Insights from a rural population laboratory. *American Journal of Epidemiology, 148,* 949–957.

Pi-Sunyer, F. X. (1993). Medical hazards of obesity. *Annals of Internal Medicine, 119*(7 pt. 2), 655–660.

Polivy, J. (1996). Psychological consequences of food restriction. *Journal of the American Dietetic Association, 96,* 589–592.

Radimer, K. L., Olson, C. M., Greene, J. C., Campbell, C. C., & Habicht, J-P. (1992). Understanding hunger and developing indicators to assess it in women and children. *Journal of Nutrition Education, 24*(1), 36S–45S.

Rothacker, D. Q., & Blackburn, G. L. (2000). Obesity prevalence by age group and 5-year changes in adults residing in rural Wisconsin. *Journal of the American Dietetic Association, 100,* 784–790.

Rural Families Speak (2002). About Rural Families Speak. Retrieved April 2, 2003, from http://www.rural families.umn.edu/about.htm

Sobal, J. (1999). Sociological analysis of the stigmatisation of obesity. In J. Germov & L. Williams (Eds.), *A sociology of food and nutrition: The social appetite.* Oxford, England: Oxford University Press.

Sobal, J., Troiano, R. P., & Frongillo, E. A., Jr. (1996). Rural-urban differences in obesity. *Rural Sociology, 61,* 289–305.

Strauss, A. L., & Corbin, J. (1990). *Basics of qualitative research: Grounded theory procedures and techniques.* Newbury Park, CA: Sage.

Tai-Seale, T., & Chandler, C. (2003). Nutrition and overweight concerns in rural areas. In L. D. Gamm, L. L. Hutchison, B. J. Dabney, & A. M. Dorsey (Eds.), *Rural healthy people 2010: A companion document to Healthy People 2010.* College Station, TX: The Texas A&M University System Health Science Center, School of Rural Public Health, Southwest Rural Health Research Center.

Townsend, M. S., Peerson, J., Love, B., Achterberg, C., & Murphy, S. P. (2001). Food insecurity is positively related to overweight in women. *Journal of Nutrition, 131*, 1738–1745.

Chapter 5

Preterm Delivery and Low Birthweight Among Rural Women: The Importance of the Preconception Physical and Mental Health Status

Marianne M. Hillemeier, Carol S. Weisman, Gary A. Chase, and Megan Romer

Preterm birth (delivery prior to 37 weeks of gestation) and low birthweight (less than 2500 grams or 5 pounds 8 ounces) are interrelated pregnancy outcomes that greatly increase the chances of infant death in the first year of life and predispose the infants who survive to chronic health problems and developmental disabilities (Goldenberg & Rouse, 1998; Paneth 1995). Reducing the occurrence

The authors are indebted to Chris Hollenbeak, PhD, who conducted the analyses of hospitalization data from the Pennsylvania Health Care Cost Containment Council. The authors are grateful to the Pennsylvania Department of Health for providing access to birth registration data for counties in the study region. The CePAWHS project is funded, in part, under a grant with the Pennsylvania Department of Health. The Department specifically disclaims responsibility for any analyses, interpretations, or conclusions drawn by the authors or researchers.

of these adverse pregnancy outcomes is a high-priority public health goal, highlighted by the Centers for Disease Control and Prevention in its *Healthy People 2010* initiative (U.S. Department of Health and Human Services [USDHHS], 2000), as well as in a related effort, *Rural Healthy People 2010* (Gamm, Hutchison, Dabney, & Dorsey, 2003). These outcomes also represent some of the most serious and persistent examples of health disparities associated with race/ethnicity, socioeconomic status, and geographic location. Nationally, about 20 percent of births occur among rural women, although less attention has been paid to births in rural areas compared with more urbanized areas.

This chapter provides an overview of the problem of preterm birth and low birthweight among rural women, discusses risk factors that are of particular concern among rural women, and describes an innovative new approach to prevention, the Central Pennsylvania Women's Health Study (CePAWHS) Project. This project, involving a large, population-based cohort of women in Central Pennsylvania, focuses on the importance of women's physical and mental health *prior to pregnancy* in determining their subsequent risks for preterm birth and low birthweight.

SCOPE OF THE PROBLEM

Despite considerable research effort and policy attention, preterm birth rates in the United States have increased in recent years, and currently over 12 percent of all deliveries are less than fullterm (Martin et al., 2003). Growth in the number of twin and higher-order multiple pregnancies, primarily due to assisted reproductive technology and increasing average age at pregnancy, is a contributing factor, since multiple pregnancies are more prone to early delivery (Blondel et al., 2002). However, the rate of preterm birth among single pregnancies is also on the rise (Alexander & Slay, 2002). As a consequence, the proportion of infants born with low birthweight has increased, and the current rate of 7.8 percent is the highest level reported in over three decades (Martin et al., 2003).

Over four million infants are born in the U.S. each year, and about 20 percent of those births are to rural mothers (Lishner, Larson, Rosenblatt, & Clark, 1999). Analyses of national data suggest that, overall, crude rates of low birthweight in nonmetropolitan areas are slightly lower than rates in metropolitan areas, although they are not significantly different after socioeconomic and health care factors have been taken into account (Peck & Alexander, 2003). Rural-urban patterns of low birthweight have been found to vary importantly by race. White women, who account for the majority of births in both rural and urban settings, and those who live in nonmetropolitan counties have consistently higher rates of low birthweight compared with those living in metropolitan counties (Lishner et al., 1999; Larson, Hart, & Rosenblatt, 1997). Nonmetropolitan African American and American Indian women, in contrast, have lower rates of low birthweight than their urban counterparts (Lishner et al., 1999; Larson, Hart, & Rosenblatt, 1997).

Improvements in access to prenatal care since the 1980s, largely due to Medicaid expansions, have not been accompanied by a decline in indicators of adverse pregnancy outcomes, nor have disparities in these outcomes been reduced (Frick & Lantz, 1999; Lu & Halfon, 2003). A recent evidence review of the effectiveness of prenatal care for preventing low birthweight concluded that neither preterm birth nor intrauterine growth restriction (the two key determinants of low birthweight) could be prevented by prenatal care in its present form (Lu, Alexander, Kotelchuck, & Halfon, 2003). Skepticism is mounting about the efficacy of interventions targeted at women who are already pregnant (Grason, Hutchins, & Silver, 1999; Kotelchuck, 2003; Wise, 2003). Thus, although increasing access to early and adequate prenatal care remains an important goal, particularly among rural populations where access to health care is more limited than in urbanized areas, this alone is not expected to reduce disparities in preterm birth and low birthweight.

RISK FACTORS FOR PRETERM BIRTH AND LOW BIRTHWEIGHT AMONG RURAL WOMEN

The causal mechanisms underlying early delivery and low birthweight are not well understood (Slattery & Morrison, 2002; Goldenberg & Rouse, 1998). Epidemiological studies, however, have identified factors that tend to be associated with these outcomes (Alexander & Slay, 2002), many of which are common among rural women and are likely to increase their risk. For example, socioeconomic disadvantage has been consistently associated with an increased likelihood of preterm birth and low birthweight (Parker, Schoendorf, & Kiely, 1994; Kogan, 1995; Kramer, Séguin, Lydon, & Goelet, 2000; Finch, 2003). Rural poverty rates are nearly 20 percent higher than urban rates, and currently 14.2 percent of those outside metropolitan areas live in poverty (DeNavas-Walt, Proctor, & Mills, 2004). The poverty rate is highest in completely rural counties, where 16.8 percent of the population is poor (Jolliffe, 2004). The median income of rural households was $35,112 in 2003, as compared with $46,060 in metropolitan areas (DeNavas-Walt, Proctor, & Mills, 2004), reflecting fewer employment opportunities and lower educational levels (Whitener & McGranahan, 2003). Although educational attainment among rural residents continues to rise, only about 15 percent of nonmetropolitan adults age 25 and over have graduated from a four-year college and only three-quarters of adults have a high school diploma or GED equivalent (Gibbs, 2004).

Rural women are also disproportionately likely to experience health risks that can increase their chances for poor pregnancy outcomes. Nationally, adults living in rural areas are the most likely to smoke, with current rates among rural women above one in four (Eberhardt et al., 2001). Obesity, which is linked to poor birth outcomes through its association with diabetes, heart disease, and other chronic illnesses, is most prevalent in rural counties, with a self-reported rate in the most rural counties approaching 25 percent (Eberhardt et al., 2001). Toxic exposures to herbicides and pesticides that can adversely impact pregnancy outcome are also more common in rural areas, where farm workers may inadvertently expose family members via pesticide residues on their skin and clothing (Goldman, Eskenazi, Bradman, & Jewell, 2004; Gaston, 2001). High levels of psychosocial stress may also be common among rural women, related in part to lack of material resources, geographic isolation, social pressure to conform with predominantly conservative lifestyle choices, and uncertainty associated with a livelihood tied to agriculture (Mulder et al., 1999; Bushy, 1998)

Health risks among rural women are further exacerbated by reduced access to appropriate medical care. Both health care providers—especially medical specialists—and high-quality medical facilities are less likely to be located in rural areas (Hart, Lishner, &

Rosenblatt, 2003; Larsen & Fleishman, 2003), and their lower income and employment levels make it more difficult for rural women to maintain health insurance coverage (Ziller, Coburn, Loux, Hoffman, & McBride, 2003). With regard to health care utilization, rural women receive fewer screening and preventive services (Casey, Call, & Klingner, 2001), receive less adequate prenatal care (Peck & Alexander, 2003), and make fewer ambulatory care visits than women in more urbanized areas (Larson, Machlin, Nixon, & Zodet, 2004). Fragmentation of women's health care may be exacerbated in rural areas, due in part to the relative scarcity of obstetrician-gynecologists and to fewer resources with which to establish comprehensive women's health care programs (Eberhardt et al., 2001). Problems in obtaining transportation to medical care facilities (Friedman, 2004; Agency for Healthcare Research and Quality [AHRQ], 1996), as well as lack of knowledge about the importance of preventive medical care contribute to rural women's suboptimal utilization of health services. It has also been suggested that rural cultural values including self-sufficiency, belief in traditional social roles for women, and reluctance to seek medical care unless seriously ill play a role in decreased utilization of health care services among rural women (Casey, Call, & Klingner, 2001; Hauenstein, 2003; Mulder et al., 1999; Larson & Fleishman, 2003).

CONCEPTUALIZING THE MECHANISMS UNDERLYING PRETERM BIRTH AND LOW BIRTHWEIGHT

Although a comprehensive theory of the determinants of preterm birth and low birthweight is not available, Misra, Guyer, and Allston (2003) have provided an "integrated perinatal health framework" that takes a lifespan perspective on reproductive health, rather than focusing only on pregnancy. This framework classifies risk factors for adverse pregnancy outcomes based on the Evans and Stoddart (1990) model of multiple health determinants. This classification distinguishes between *distal* and *proximal* determinants of health. Distal determinants affect susceptibility to proximal determinants and include genetic factors, the physical environment, and the social or community environment. Proximal determinants include the biomedical and behavioral responses of individuals that affect outcomes.

The lifespan perspective incorporated into Misra and colleagues' (2003) model affects how distal and proximal determinants are conceptualized and measured. For example, psychosocial stress is considered to be both acute and chronic, with effects on health that accumulate over time. This is consistent with the *weathering* process proposed by Geronimus (2001), whereby women's health reflects the cumulative impact of life experiences, including psychosocial stressors, from conception to the present. Health care (including public health programs, health information, and personal medical care) modifies relationships among variables in the model. Misra and colleagues (2003) argue that the proximal risks for adverse pregnancy outcomes are key targets for interventions in the preconceptional and interconceptional periods. A life-course perspective and greater investment in the health of women also have been proposed by scholars concerned about the persistence of racial/ethnic disparities in birth outcomes (Lu & Halfon, 2003).

For the CePAWHS project, which is described in detail in the next section, risk factors are classified as shown in Figure 5.1. This framework is adapted from Misra and colleagues (2003) to guide the project, which has preterm birth and low birthweight outcomes as endpoints. The focus is on women's preconceptional health, including chronic conditions, infections, and psychosocial stress and stress-related behavior as proximal risk factors. Pregnancy-specific factors such as preeclampsia and prior adverse pregnancy outcomes are also included. The risk factors in each preconceptional health category have been identified in previous studies of preterm birth and low birthweight as discussed below, although some have been subjected to less research than others.

Psychosocial Stress and Stress-Related Behavior

Psychosocial stress has long been considered as a risk factor in preterm birth and low birthweight (e.g., Nuckolls, Kaplan, & Cassell, 1972), although early methodologically limited studies yielded inconclusive findings (Hogue, Hoffman, & Hatch, 2001). More recently, associations have been reported between preterm birth and both acute and chronic stressors, including stressful life events, stressful

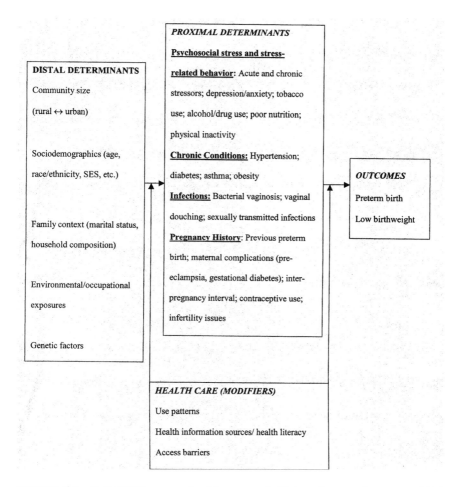

FIGURE 5.1 CePAWHS conceptual framework: Determinants of preterm birth and low birthweight.

work, physical abuse, racism, smoking, alcohol and drug use, poor nutrition, physical inactivity, low levels of social support during pregnancy, anxiety, and depression (Copper et al., 1996; Dole et al., 2003; Dunkel-Schetter, 1998; Hobel & Culhane, 2003; Leiferman & Evenson, 2003; Mamelle, Measson, Munoz, & Audreas de la Bastie, 1998; Misra, O'Campo, & Strobino, 2001; Misra, Guyer, & Alston, 2003; Mutale, Creed, Maresh, & Hunt, 1991; Nordentoft et al., 1996; Orr et al., 1996; Orr, James, & Blackmore Prince, 2002; Rich-Edwards et al., 2001). The disproportionate risk for these stressors among poor, rural, and minority women, coupled with increasing evidence about the biological plausibility of stress-related mechanisms of preterm labor (Wadhwa et al., 2001), suggest that further exploration of stress-related interventions before pregnancy is needed.

Chronic Conditions

The prevalence of chronic disease is disproportionately greater among poor and minority women (Ephraim, Misra, Nguyen, & Vahratian, 2001; Geronimus, 2001) and many chronic conditions increase the risk of giving birth prematurely and of having a low-birthweight infant (Misra, Grason, & Weisman, 2000). Chronic hypertension is associated with both preterm birth and low birthweight (Sibai, 2002), with minority women at disproportionately greater risk (Barton, Barton, O'Brien, Berganer, & Sibai, 2002). Preexisting insulin dependent diabetes mellitus is associated with increased incidence of preterm delivery (Wylie et al., 2002), particularly among women whose diabetes is in poor control (Sibai et al., 2000). Women with asthma have a greater risk of both preterm birth and low birthweight, as well as adverse maternal outcomes, including preeclampsia, chorioamnionitis, and cesarean delivery (Liu, Wen, Demissie, Marcoux, & Kramer, 2001). Maternal obesity adversely impacts pregnancy outcomes, primarily through increased rates of hypertension, diabetes, and infection, which elevate preterm delivery risk (Castro & Avina, 2002).

Infections

Maternal urogenital tract infection is an important risk factor for preterm birth (Romero et al., 2001; Wadhwa et al., 2001). The presence of bacterial vaginosis (BV) at any time in pregnancy has been found to be associated with an approximately twofold increase in the risk of preterm labor and premature rupture of membranes, and the risk increases more than sevenfold when BV is detected early in pregnancy (Andrews, Hauth, & Goldenberg, 2000; Hillier et al., 1995; Leitich et al., 2003). Intrauterine infection is implicated as a key factor in up to 40 percent of preterm deliveries, with higher prevalence rates among disadvantaged and minority women as well

TABLE 5.1 Birth Outcomes and Maternal Risk Characteristics by Mother's County of Residence, 2002, in Comparison With Healthy People 2010 Goals

County	Pre-term Birth Rate[a]	Low Birth Weight Rate[b]	Very Low Birth Weight Rate[c]	1st Trimester Prenatal Care	Non-Smoking Mothers	Chronic High Blood Pressure	Pregnancy-Induced High Blood Pressure	Any Diabetes
Healthy People 2010 Goals	7.60	5.00	0.90	90.00	99.00	–	–	–
Adams	8.32	7.29	1.74	83.69	85.31	0.44	4.68	2.18
Bedford	7.79	5.88	0.95	86.15	81.59	0.57	4.55	6.07
Blair	8.48	7.21	1.30	91.90	75.63	0.55	3.09	5.77
Bradford	4.92	3.53	0.46	86.68	74.39	0.61	4.60	3.37
Cambria	9.22	8.44	1.38	89.71	77.95	0.83	4.70	5.18
Centre	7.11	5.84	1.44	87.92	87.79	0.88	4.15	6.70
Clinton	8.57	6.90	1.43	84.99	77.38	1.67	12.62	4.76
Columbia	10.72	7.96	2.14	82.06	80.40	2.76	7.04	5.82
Cumberland	9.52	8.31	1.38	90.41	86.70	1.19	5.51	4.18
Dauphin	10.20	10.75	1.79	90.58	87.98	1.24	3.52	2.64
Franklin	9.92	6.27	1.71	83.63	80.90	1.43	5.35	3.64
Fulton	8.40	6.72	0.00	80.51	78.15	4.20	3.36	4.20
Huntingdon	10.48	7.55	1.05	87.50	79.66	0.63	4.61	2.94
Juniata	7.03	5.81	1.53	76.32	84.40	1.22	4.59	4.59

(continued)

TABLE 5.1 *(continued)*

County	Pre-term Birth Rate[a]	Low Birth Weight Rate[b]	Very Low Birth Weight Rate[c]	1st Trimester Prenatal Care	Non-Smoking Mothers	Chronic High Blood Pressure	Pregnancy-Induced High Blood Pressure	Any Diabetes
Lancaster	7.75	6.18	1.01	78.59	87.75	0.94	4.19	4.37
Lebanon	8.67	6.93	1.64	81.84	83.85	0.52	2.75	2.09
Lycoming	9.88	7.09	1.54	80.89	75.73	0.85	4.70	4.62
Mifflin	7.36	5.51	1.17	72.77	81.64	1.17	2.84	2.84
Montour	9.59	6.82	1.36	85.85	80.91	2.73	6.82	5.45
Northumberland	9.95	7.54	1.15	86.13	75.71	1.78	5.65	6.28
Perry	9.55	7.31	1.73	84.58	81.54	1.92	5.00	3.08
Potter	6.29	4.00	0.57	94.26	68.57	2.86	8.00	4.57
Snyder	8.45	7.53	1.60	75.95	86.99	0.91	5.48	6.39
Somerset	9.10	6.42	0.80	87.72	79.95	0.80	2.54	2.54
Sullivan	7.84	11.54	1.92	80.00	78.85	1.92	1.92	3.85
Tioga	4.48	3.91	0.28	87.61	79.33	1.96	6.15	3.35
Union	9.07	6.68	0.95	74.24	87.35	2.15	4.06	8.11
York	9.99	8.15	1.63	86.36	80.06	0.98	4.6	4.6

[a]Percentage of live births < 37 weeks of gestation
[b]Percentage of live births < 2,500 grams
[c]Percentage of live births < 1,500 grams
Note: n = 33,025 live births in 28 central Pennsylvania counties

as younger women generally (Goldenberg et al., 1996; Hillier et al., 1995; Meis et al., 1995). Both BV and sexually transmitted infections (STIs) are important components of women's health that have not been addressed adequately. The relationship among infection, immunity, and stress requires further investigation (Hobel & Culhane, 2003). The practice of vaginal douching, which is prevalent in some adolescent and African American populations, has been linked with genital tract infections and may increase the risk of preterm birth (Fiscella, Franks, Kendrick, Meldrum, & Kieke, 2002; Foch, McDaniel, & Chacko, 2001; Holzman, Leventhal, Qiu, Jones, & Wang, 2001; Ness et al., 2002).

The multiplicity of risks for preterm birth and low birthweight has two implications for research. First, data available from birth registry data, hospital discharge and managed care data sets, and ongoing surveys such as the Behavioral Risk Factor Surveillance System (BRFSS) and the National Health and Nutrition Examination Survey (NHANES) provide prevalence estimates for only a limited number of risks. A more comprehensive risk profile for rural women is needed. Second, the range of risk factors for preterm birth and low birthweight implies that a single-factor intervention is not likely to be effective. Interventions should address multiple risks, be tailored to the needs of high-risk groups, and address multiple levels (e.g., consumers, health care providers, communities). For example, an intervention focusing on preconceptional screening and treatment of bacterial vaginosis or other infections would have to address women's awareness of BV and access to health care providers in addition to the technical aspects of clinical treatment.

THE CEPAWHS PROJECT

The CePAWHS project was designed to address the need for both comprehensive information on the health status of rural women and a multilevel intervention approach to reduction of preterm birth and low birthweight. It includes 1) a population-based survey of reproductive-aged women; and 2) a multidimensional intervention designed to promote the health of high-risk women prior to pregnancy.

Target Population

The CePAWHS project focuses on a 28-county region in central Pennsylvania that includes a large rural population. According to the 2000 U.S. Census, 23 percent of Pennsylvania is designated as rural: the target region contains 15 counties whose populations are predominantly or entirely rural (Adams, Bedford, Bradford, Clinton, Fulton, Huntingdon, Juniata, Mifflin, Montour, Perry, Potter, Snyder, Somerset, Sullivan, and Tioga). This region accounted for 24 percent of all births in Pennsylvania in 2001. Birth record data for 2002 show that nearly all of the counties in this region have low birthweight rates that are considerably higher than the *Healthy People 2010* goal, and 23 of the 28 counties have preterm birth rates greater than the *Healthy People* target. All but four counties in the study region fail to meet the *Healthy People 2010* goal for first trimester initiation of prenatal care. Birth certificate data related to maternal health status indicate that chronic high blood pressure and diabetes are important health concerns among women in many of the target counties. Rates of smoking during pregnancy are also high, reaching 25–30 percent in a number of rural counties.

The costs associated with preterm birth and low birthweight in this region are considerable. Hospital charges alone are high and increasing. According to data from the Pennsylvania Health Care Cost Containment Council, of the 33,541 hospital-based births in this region in 2002, 8.4 percent were premature, 5.8 percent were low birthweight, and 1.6 percent were very low birthweight (under 1500 grams or 3.3 pounds). The average hospital charges in this region were $1,212 for normal births; $35,478 for premature births; $19,291 for low birthweight births; and $104,537 for very low birthweight births.

This region is relatively disadvantaged in terms of socioeconomic status indicators and health care resources, as shown in Table 5.2.

According to the 2000 U.S. Census, 19 of the counties had median household incomes below the state median ($40,106), and 14 of the counties had higher percentages of persons in poverty than the state overall (11.0 percent). In the Pennsylvania population as a whole, 81.4 percent of those 25 years and older were high school graduates, while 22 of the 28 counties in the study region had lower

TABLE 5.2 Socioeconomic and Health Care Characteristics of 28 Central Pennsylvania Counties

County	% Rural Population[a]	Median Household Income, 1999	% Below Poverty Level, 1999[b]	% High School Grads (age 25+), 1999	Number of Hospitals Providing Obstetric Care, 2001	Number of Hospitals With NICU, 2001	Primary Care, Office-Based MDs per 100,000 Population, 2001	Ob-Gyns per 100,000 Population, 2001
Adams	60	$42,704	7.1	79.7	1	0	78.87	3.29
Bedford	84	$32,731	10.3	78.3	1	0	50.02	6.00
Blair	26	$32,861	12.6	83.8	4	0	186.61	16.26
Bradford	72	$35,038	11.8	81.7	2	0	258.12	11.15
Cambria	32	$30,179	12.5	80.0	2	2	184.80	9.17
Centre	36	$36,165	18.8	88.2	1	0	158.37	9.58
Clinton	51	$31,064	14.2	80.4	1	0	79.13	2.64
Columbia	44	$34,094	13.1	80.6	2	0	113.79	10.91
Cumberland	25	$46,707	6.6	86.1	2	1	207.79	14.51
Dauphin	15	$41,507	9.7	83.4	2	2	253.38	17.47
Franklin	47	$40,476	7.6	78.9	2	0	118.32	9.28
Fulton	100	$34,882	10.8	73.2	0	0	35.06	7.01
Huntingdon	69	$33,313	11.3	74.6	1	0	87.75	4.39
Juniata	85	$34,698	9.5	74.5	0	0	17.53	0.00

(continued)

TABLE 5.2 *(continued)*

County	% Rural Population[a]	Median Household Income, 1999	% Below Poverty Level, 1999[b]	% High School Grads (age 25+), 1999	Number of Hospitals Providing Obstetric Care, 2001	Number of Hospitals With NICU, 2001	Primary Care, Office-Based MDs per 100,000 Population, 2001	Ob-Gyns per 100,000 Population, 2001
Lancaster	25	$45,507	7.8	77.4	3	1	128.33	6.37
Lebanon	36	$40,838	7.5	78.6	1	0	140.45	11.63
Lycoming	36	$34,016	11.5	80.6	1	0	144.95	6.66
Mifflin	56	$32,175	12.5	77.2	1	0	133.37	6.45
Montour	54	$38,075	8.7	82.3	1	1	1069.31	54.84
Northumberland	37	$31,314	11.9	77.8	1	0	67.68	2.12
Perry	86	$41,909	7.7	79.9	0	0	29.82	0.00
Potter	100	$32,253	12.7	80.6	1	0	110.62	5.53
Snyder	71	$35,981	9.9	73.2	0	0	61.26	5.33
Somerset	75	$30,911	11.8	77.5	2	0	83.73	5.00
Sullivan	100	$30,279	14.5	78.0	0	0	30.51	0.00
Tioga	84	$32,020	13.5	80.5	1	0	99.10	0.00
Union	45	$40,336	8.8	73.1	0	0	197.00	12.01
York	29	$45,268	6.7	80.7	3	1	124.16	7.60

[a]Census classification of "rural"
[b]Poverty rates are determined for residents in each county at the time of the 2000 Census, including students residing on college campuses.

educational attainment rates. While eight counties are home to hospitals that offer both obstetric and neonatal intensive care services, the majority lack one or the other type of hospital facilities, and 6 rural counties (Fulton, Juniata, Perry, Snyder, Sullivan, and Union) have no hospitals offering either type of service. Similarly, physician-to-population ratios indicate that relatively fewer physicians in both primary care and obstetrics-gynecology have practices located in these counties. According to the Pennsylvania Department of Health, the region also includes health professional shortage areas, defined as service areas with a critical shortage of primary care providers, and medically underserved areas, defined as areas or populations with a shortage of health care services in addition to selected health and population factors.

The target region contains ethnically diverse communities, with county populations ranging from 75.6 percent to 98.2 percent White, non-Hispanic. The region includes populations of African Americans primarily in the Harrisburg area, Latinas in the Lancaster area (traditional Mennonite and Amish communities), and various immigrant communities.

Community Survey

The first phase of the CePAWHS project is a population-based survey to determine the prevalence of risk factors for preterm birth and low birthweight and the relationships among risk factors and race/ethnicity, socioeconomic status, rural residence, and women's health care access and utilization patterns. This survey will consist of several components: (1) a telephone survey, using random-digit dialing (RDD), with a representative sample of 2,000 reproductive-age women (ages 18–45) residing in the target region; (2) household interviews of an additional 300 women (ages 18–45) residing in traditional Amish communities that do not have household telephones; and (3) interviews with 300 adolescents (ages 16–17) in family planning clinics. This survey is unique in studies of preterm birth and low birthweight outcomes because it is based on a representative community sample rather than a sample of clinically ascertained pregnant women.

Survey items address the following topic areas:

Pregnancy History

This includes measures of prior pregnancies and births; prior preterm or low birthweight births; maternal complications during pregnancy; and interpregnancy interval.

Health Status

This includes measures of chronic conditions and infections diagnosed by a doctor, using items from national surveys of women's health; a short-form depressive symptoms scale based on the CES-D instrument (Radloff, 1977) from the Commonwealth Fund Survey of Women's Health (Collins et al., 1999); overall health and disability status based on scales in the SF-12 instrument (Ware & Sherbourne, 1992); and height and weight for computing body mass index.

Psychosocial Stress

This includes measures of acute and chronic stressors from studies of preterm birth and low birthweight (Dole et al., 2003; Misra, O'Campo, & Strobino, 2001); survey measures of exposure to domestic or intimate partner violence adapted from the Commonwealth Fund Survey of Women's Health (Collins et al., 1999); and perceptions of discrimination based on race/ethnicity and gender.

Health Behaviors

This includes measures of smoking, alcohol/drug use, nutrition and physical activity, current contraceptive use, and vaginal douching, based on measures from the Behavioral Risk Factor Surveillance Survey, the National Health and Nutrition Examination Survey, and other behavioral research.

Health Care Access and Utilization

This includes measures from the Commonwealth Fund Survey of Women's Health (Collins et al., 1999) and the Kaiser Women's Health Survey (Kaiser Family Foundation, 2002) of type(s) of health insurance, usual source(s) of care, receipt of selected primary and preventive services in the past year, and access barriers such as transportation needs and lack of culturally sensitive care.

Sociodemographics

This includes measures of age, marital status, household composition, race/ethnicity, educational level, employment status, household income, and religiosity. Geocoding will permit linking individual data with community characteristics (such as race/ethnic composition, percent living in poverty, unemployment rates, and rurality) and area medical resources (such as presence of a hospital providing obstetrical services, ratio of obstetrician-gynecologists and other primary care providers to population).

Intervention

The conceptual framework guiding this project (see Figure 5.1) provides the rationale for a multidimensional intervention targeting prevalent risk factors in preconceptional women. The survey described above will document the prevalent risk factors and high-risk populations in the target region. The intervention will target key proximal risk factors and will be tested in diverse populations at risk, with particular attention to identifying opportunities for interventions in rural populations. The intervention is planned to incorporate the following attributes:

- It targets the *preconceptional* (and interconceptional) period.

- It is *population-based* (i.e., it is based on population-level data and will be implemented with women recruited in community as well as clinical settings, in order to ensure participation by women who do not have regular health care access or reside in rural areas).

- It is *multidimensional* (i.e., it addresses multiple biopsychosocial risks for preterm birth and low birthweight).

- It targets *multiple health outcomes* (i.e., health knowledge/ literacy, self-efficacy, health behavior change, access to health care, and health status).

- It is offered in *group sessions* (rather than one on one).

- It is *multilevel* in that (1) the information and skills provided are relevant both to individual health behaviors and to interpersonal relationships and social factors affecting health; (2)

students in health care professions will be trained to facilitate the intervention sessions; and (3) information about the intervention content will be disseminated to primary care providers in the community.

- It is *evidence-based* in that the content of the intervention depends upon the findings of the population-based survey.

CONCLUSION

Preterm birth and low birthweight are high-priority pregnancy outcomes that greatly elevate the risk of mortality in the first year of life, increase the likelihood that infants who survive will experience morbidity and disability often persisting into adulthood, and account for an important share of current health-care costs. Although about one of every five infants is born to a rural mother, salient risk factors for preterm birth and low birthweight in this population are not well understood.

The CePAWHS project addresses the need for in-depth information on the health status of rural women and their risks for adverse pregnancy outcomes through a comprehensive, population-based survey that assesses both reproductive history and underlying physical and mental health status. Findings from the survey will form the basis of an innovative, multilevel intervention to reduce preterm birth and low birthweight among rural women through the reduction of health risks prior to pregnancy. This project offers the opportunity to advance our understanding of the mechanisms underlying these adverse pregnancy outcomes, as well as to promote improvements in the wellbeing of rural women and the health chances of their infants.

REFERENCES

Agency for Healthcare Research and Quality (1996). Improving Health Care for Rural Populations. AHCPR Publication No. 96-P040. Retrieved October 4, 2004, from http://www.ahrq.gov/research/rural.htm

Alexander, G. R., & Slay, M. (2002). Prematurity at birth: Trends, racial disparities, and epidemiology. *Mental Retardation and Developmental Disabilities Research Review, 8*(4), 215–220.

Andrews, W. W., Hauth, J. C., & Goldenberg, R. L. (2000). Infection and preterm birth. *American Journal of Perinatology, 17*(7), 357–365.

Barton, C. B., Barton, J. R., O'Brien, J. M., Berganer, N. K., & Sibai, B. M. (2002). Mild gestational hypertension: Differences in ethnicity are associated with altered outcomes in women who undergo outpatient treatment. *American Journal of Obstetrics and Gynecology, 186*(5), 896–898.

Blondel, B., Kogan, M. D., Alexander, G. R., Dattani, N., Kramer, M. S., Macfarlane, A., et al. (2002). The impact of the increasing number of multiple births on the rates of preterm birth and low birthweight: An international study. *American Journal of Public Health, 92*(8), 1323–1330.

Bushy, A. (1998). Health issues of women in rural environments: an overview. *Journal of the American Medical Women's Association, 53*(2), 53–56.

Casey, M. M., Call, K. T., & Klingner, J. M. (2001). Are rural residents less likely to obtain recommended preventive healthcare services? *American Journal of Preventive Medicine, 21*(3), 182–188.

Castro, L. C., & Avina, R. L. (2002). Maternal obesity and pregnancy outcomes. *Current Opinion in Obstetrics and Gynecology, 14*(6), 601–606.

Collins, K. S., Schoen, C., Joseph, S., Duchon, L., Simantov, E., & Yellowitz, M. (1999). *Health concerns across a woman's lifespan: The Commonwealth Fund 1998 Survey of Women's Health*. New York: The Commonwealth Fund.

Copper, R. L., Goldenberg, R. L., Das, A., Elder, N., Swain, M., Norman, G., et al. (1996). The preterm prediction study: Maternal stress is associated with spontaneous preterm birth at less than thirty-five weeks' gestation. *American Journal of Obstetrics and Gynecology, 175*(5), 1286–1292.

DeNavas-Walt, C., Proctor, B. D., & Mills, R. J. (2004). Income, poverty, and health insurance coverage in the United States: 2003. Current Population Reports, P60–226. Washington, DC: U.S. Government Printing Office.

Dole, N., Savitz, D. A., Hertz-Picciotto, I., Siega-Riz, A. M., McMahon, M. J., & Buekens, P. (2003). Maternal stress and preterm birth. *American Journal of Epidemiology, 157*(1), 14–24.

Dunkel-Schetter, C. (1998). Maternal stress and preterm delivery. *Prenatal and Neonatal Medicine, 3*, 39–42.

Eberhardt, M. S., Ingram, D. D., Makuc, D. M., Pamuk, E. R., Freid, V. M., Harper, S. B., et al. (2001). Urban and Rural Health Chartbook: Health, United States. Hyattsville, MD: National Center for Health Statistics.

Ephraim, P., Misra, D., Nguyen, R., & Vahratian, A. (2001). Chronic conditions. In D. Misra (Ed.), *The women's health data book* (3rd ed.). Washington, DC: Jacobs Institute of Women's Health and Henry J. Kaiser Family Foundation.

Evans, R. G., & Stoddart, G. L. (1990). Producing health, consuming health care. *Social Science and Medicine, 31*(12), 1347–1363.

Finch, B. K. (2003). Socioeconomic gradients and low birth-weight: Empirical and policy considerations. *Health Services Research, 38*(6p1), 1819–1841.

Fiscella, K., Franks, P., Kendrick, J. S., Meldrum, S., & Kieke, B. A. (2002). Risk of preterm birth that is associated with vaginal douching. *American Journal of Obstetrics and Gynecology, 186*(6), 1345–1350.

Foch, B. J., McDaniel, N. D., & Chacko, M. R. (2001). Racial differences in vaginal douching knowledge, attitude, and practices among sexually active adolescents. *Journal of Pediatric and Adolescent Gynecology, 14*(1), 29–33.

Frick, K. D., & Lantz, P. M. (1999). How well do we understand the relationship between prenatal care and birth weight? *Health Services Research, 34*(5p1), 1063–1073.

Friedman, P. (2004). Transportation needs in rural communities. Rural Assistance Center Issue Note, 2(1). Retrieved October 4, 2004 from http://www.raconline.org/infor_guides/transportation/issuenote.html

Gamm, L. D., Hutchison, L., Dabney, B. J., & Dorsey, A. M. (2003). *Rural Healthy People 2010: A Companion Document to Healthy People 2010*, Vol. 2. College Station, TX: Texas A&M University System Health Science Center.

Gaston, M. H. (2001). 100% access and 0 health disparities: Changing the health paradigm for rural women in the 21st century. *Women's Health Issues, 11*(1), 7–16.

Geronimus, A. T. (2001). Understanding and eliminating racial inequalities in women's health in the United States: The role of the weathering conceptual framework. *Journal of the American Medical Women's Association, 56*(4), 149–150.

Gibbs, R. (2004). Rural Education at a Glance. Rural Development Research Report No. (RDRR98). Retrieved October 4, 2004 from http://www.ers.usda.gov/publications/RDRR98/

Goldenberg, R. L., Thom, E., Moawad, A. H., Johnson, F., Roberts, J., & Caritis, S. N. (1996). The preterm prediction study: Fetal fibronectin, bacterial vaginosis, and peripartum infection. National Institute of Child Health and Human Development (NICHD) Maternal Fetal Medicine Units Network. *Obstetrics & Gynecology, 87*(5), 656–660.

Goldenberg, R. L., & Rouse, D. J. (1998). Prevention of premature birth. *New England Journal of Medicine, 339*(5), 313–320.

Goldman, L., Eskenazi, B., Bradman, A., & Jewell, N. P. (2004). Risk behaviors for pesticide exposure among pregnant women living in farmworker households in Salinas, California. *American Journal of Industrial Medicine, 45*(6), 491–499.

Grason, H., Hutchins, J., & Silver, G. (Eds). (1999). *Charting a course for the future of women's and perinatal health, Vol. II.* Baltimore, MD: Women's and Children's Health Policy Center, Johns Hopkins School of Public Health.

Hart, L. G., Lishner, D. M., & Rosenblatt, R. A. (2003). Rural health workforce: Context, trends, and issues. In E. H. Larson, K. E. Johnson, T. E. Norris, D. M. Lishner, R. A. Rosenblatt, & L. G. Hart (Eds.), *State of the health workforce in rural America: Profiles and comparisons*. Seattle, WA: WWAMI Rural Health Research Center, University of Washington.

Hauenstein, E. J. (2003). No comfort in the rural south: Women living depressed. *Archives of Psychiatric Nursing, 17*(1), 3–11.

Hillier, S. L., Nugent, R. P., Eschenbach, D. A., Krohn, M. A., Gibbs, R. S., Martin, D. H., et al. (1995). Association between bacterial vaginosis and preterm delivery of a low-birthweight infant. *New England Journal of Medicine, 333*(26), 1737–1742.

Hobel, C., & Culhane, J. (2003). Role of Psychosocial and Nutritional Stress on Poor Pregnancy Outcomes. *Journal of Nutrition, 133*(5), 1709S–1717S.

Hogue, C. J. R., Hoffman, S., & Hatch, M. C. (2001). Stress and preterm delivery: A conceptual framework. *Paediatric and Perinatal Epidemiology, 15*(S2), 30–40.

Holzman, C., Leventhal, J. M., Qiu, H., Jones, N. M., & Wang, J. (2001). Factors linked to bacterial vaginosis in nonpregnant women. *American Journal of Public Health, 91*(10), 1664–1670.

Jolliffe, D. (2004). Rural Poverty at a Glance. Rural Development Research Report No. RDRR100. Retrieved October 4, 2004 from: http://www.ers.usda.gov/publications/rdrr98/rdrr98_lowres.pdf

Kaiser Family Foundation (2002). *Women's health in the United States: Health coverage and access to care.* Menlo Park, CA: Henry J. Kaiser Family Foundation.

Kogan, M. D. (1995). Social causes of low birth weight. *Journal of the Royal Society of Medicine, 88*(11), 611–615.

Kotelchuck, M. (2003). Building on a life-course perspective in maternal and child health. *Maternal and Child Health Journal, 7*(1), 5–11.

Kramer, M. S., Séguin, L., Lydon, J., & Goulet, L. (2000). Socio-economic disparities in pregnancy outcome: Why do the poor fare so poorly? *Paediatric and Perinatal Epidemiology, 14*(3), 194–210.

Larson, E. H., Hart, L. G., & Rosenblatt, R. A. (1997). Is non-metropolitan residence a risk factor for poor birth outcome in the U.S. *Social Science and Medicine, 45*(2), 171–188.

Larson, S. L., & Fleishman, J. A. (2003). Rural-urban differences in usual source of care and ambulatory service use. *Medical Care, 41*(S7), III-65–74.

Larson, S. L., Machlin, S. R., Nixon, A., & Zodet, M. (2004). *Health Care in Urban and Rural Areas, Combined Years 1998–2000* (Publication No. 04-0001). Rockville, MD: Agency for Healthcare Research and Quality.

Leiferman, J. A., & Evenson, K. R. (2003). The effect of regular leisure physical activity on birth outcomes. *Maternal and Child Health Journal, 7*(1), 59–64.

Leitich, H., Bodner-Adler, B., Brunbauer, M., Kaider, A., Egarter, C., & Husslein, P. (2003). Bacterial vaginosis as a risk factor for preterm delivery: A meta-analysis. *American Journal of Obstetrics and Gynecology, 189*(1), 139–147.

Lishner, D. M., Larson, E. H., Rosenblatt, R. A., & Clark, S. J. (1999). Rural maternal and perinatal health. In T. C. Ricketts (Ed.), *Rural health in the United States.* New York: Oxford University Press.

Liu, S., Wen, S. W., Demissie, K., Marcoux, S., & Kramer, M. S. (2001). Maternal asthma and pregnancy outcomes: A retrospective cohort study. *American Journal of Obstetrics and Gynecology, 184*(2), 90–96.

Lu, M. C., Alexander, T. V., Kotelchuck, M., & Halfon, N. (2003). Preventing low birth weight: Is prenatal care the answer? *Journal of Maternal-Fetal Medicine, 13*(6), 362–380.

Lu, M. C., & Halfon, N. (2003). Racial and ethnic disparities in birth outcomes: A life-course perspective. *Maternal and Child Health Journal, 7*(1), 13–30.

Mamelle, N., Measson, A., Munoz, F., & Audreas de la Bastie, M. (1998). Identification of psychosocial factors in preterm birth. *Prenatal and Neonatal Medicine, 3*(1), 35–38.

Martin, J. A., Hamilton, B. E., Sutton, P. D., Ventura, S. J., Menacker, F., Munson, M. L. (2003). Births: Final data for 2002. *National Vital Statistics Report, 52*(10), 1–113.

Meis, P. J., Goldenberg, R. L., Mercer, B., Moawad, A., Das, A., McNellis, D., et al. (1995). The preterm prediction study: Significance of vaginal infections. *American Journal of Obstetrics and Gynecology, 173*(4), 1231–1235.

Misra, D. P., Grason, H., & Weisman, C. (2000). An intersection of women's and perinatal health: The role of chronic conditions. *Women's Health Issues, 10*(5), 256–267.

Misra, D. P., O'Campo, P., & Strobino, D. (2001). Testing a sociomedical model for preterm delivery. *Paediatric and Perinatal Epidemiology, 15*(2), 110–122.

Misra, D. P., Guyer, B., & Allston, A. (2003). Integrated perinatal health framework: A multiple determinants model with a life span approach. *American Journal of Preventive Medicine, 25*(1), 65–75.

Mulder, P. L., Kenkel, M. B., Shellenberger, S., Constantine, M. G., Streiegel, R., Sears, S. F. Jr., et al. (1999). The Behavioral Health Care Needs of Rural Women. Report commissioned by the American Psychological Association. Retrieved October 4, 2004 from http://www.apa.org/rural/ruralwomen.pdf

Mutale, T., Creed, F., Maresh, M., & Hunt, L. (1991). Life events and low birthweight—analysis by infants preterm and small for gestational age. *British Journal of Obstetrics and Gynaecology, 98*, 166–172.

Ness, R. B., Hillier, S. L., Richter, H. E., Soper, D. E., Stamm, C., McGregory, J., et al. (2002). Douching in relation to bacterial vaginosis, lactobacilli, and facultative bacteria in the vagina. *Obstetrics and Gynecology, 100*(4), 765–772.

Nordentoft, M., Lou, H. C., Hansen, D., Nim, J., Pryds, O., Rubin, P., et al. (1996). Intrauterine growth retardation and premature delivery: The influence of maternal smoking and psychosocial factors. *American Journal of Public Health, 86*(3), 347–354.

Nuckolls, K. B., Kaplan, B. H., & Cassell, J. (1972). Psychosocial assets, life crisis and the prognosis of pregnancy. *American Journal of Epidemiology, 95*, 431–441.

Orr, S. T., James, S. A., & Blackmore Prince, C. (2002). Maternal prenatal depressive symptoms and spontaneous preterm births among African American women in Baltimore, Maryland. *American Journal of Epidemiology, 156*(9), 797–802.

Orr, S. T., James, S. A., Miller, C. A., Barakat, B., Daikoku, N., Pupkin, M., et al. (1996). Psychosocial stressors and low birthweight in an urban population. *American Journal of Preventive Medicine, 12*(6), 459–466.

Paneth, N. S. (1995). The problem of low birthweight. *Future of Children, 5*(1), 19–34.

Parker, J. D., Schoendorf, K. C., & Kiely, J. L. (1994). Associations between measures of socioeconomic status and low birth weight, small for gestational age, and premature delivery in the United States. *Annals of Epidemiology, 4*(4), 271–278.

Peck, J., & Alexander, K. (2003). Maternal, infant, and child health in rural areas: A literature review. In L. D. Gamm, L. Hutchison, B. J. Dabney, & A. M. Dorsey

(Eds.), *Rural Healthy People 2010: A Companion Document to Healthy People 2010* (Vol. 2). College Station, TX: Texas A&M University System Health Science Center.

Radloff, L. S. (1977). The CES-D scale: A self-report depression scale for research in the general population. *Applied Psychological Measurement, 1*, 385–401.

Rich-Edwards, J., Kreiger, N., Majzoub, J., Zierler, S., Liberman, E., & Gillman, M. (2001). Maternal experiences of racism and violence as predictors of preterm birth: Rationale and Study Design. *Paediatric and Perinatal Epidemiology, 15*(S2), 124–135.

Romero, R., Gomez, R., Chaiworapongsa, T., Conoscenti, G., Kim, J. C., & Kim, Y. M. (2001). The role of infection in preterm labour and delivery. *Paediatric and Perinatal Epidemiology, 15*(S2), 41–56.

Sibai, B. M., Caritis, S., Hauth, J., Lindheimer, M., VanDorsten, J. P., MacPherson, C., et al. (2000). Risks of preeclampsia and adverse neonatal outcomes among women with pregestational diabetes mellitus. NICHD Network of Maternal-Fetal Medicine Units. *American Journal of Obstetrics and Gynecology, 182*(2), 364–369.

Sibai, B. M. (2002). Chronic hypertension in pregnancy. *Obstetrics and Gynecology, 100*(2), 369–377.

Slattery, M. M., & Morrison, J. J. (2002). Preterm delivery. *Lancet, 360*(9344), 1489–1497.

U.S. Department of Health and Human Services (2000). *Healthy People 2010: Understanding and improving health* (2nd ed.). Washington, DC: U.S. Government Printing Office.

Wadhwa, P. D., Culhane, J. F., Rauh, V., Barve, S. S., Hogan, V., Sandman, C. A., et al. (2001). Stress, infection and preterm birth: A biobehavioral perspective. *Paediatric and Perinatal Epidemiology, 15*(S2), 17–29.

Ware, J. E., & Sherbourne, C. D. (1992). The MOS 36-item short-form health survey (SF-36), I: Conceptual framework and item selection. *Medical Care, 30*(6), 473–483.

Wise, P. H. (2003). The anatomy of a disparity in infant mortality. *Annual Review of Public Health, 24*, 1–22.

Whitener, L. A., & McGranahan, D. A. (2003). Rural America: Opportunities and challenges. *Amber Waves, 1*(1), 14–21.

Wylie, B. R., Kong, J., Kozak, S. E., Marshall, C. J., Tong, S. O., & Thompson, D. M. (2002). Normal perinatal mortality in Type 1 diabetes mellitus in a series of 300 consecutive pregnancy outcomes. *American Journal of Perinatology, 19*(4), 169–176.

Ziller, E. C., Coburn, A. F., Loux, S. L., Hoffman, C., & McBride, T. D. (2003). Health Insurance Coverage in Rural America: Chartbook. Kaiser Commission on Medicaid and the Uninsured. Retrieved October 4, 2004 from http://www.kff.org/uninsured/4093.cfm

Chapter 6

Mental Health Parity Still Evading Rural Women

Jane Nelson Bolin

INTRODUCTION

The Mental Health Parity Act (MHPA), originally set to expire under sunset provisions in September 2001, has twice been extended by Congress (Center for Medicare and Medicaid Services [CMS], 2003; Department of Labor [DOL], 2003). Through piecemeal interim amendments Congress has managed to extend the MHPA in order to continue mental health treatment coverage for workers insured under group health plans under the Act. However, Congress still has not addressed the lack of mental health insurance coverage for millions of individuals who were *not* covered by the MHPA, many of whom live in rural areas, work for small employers, and work in jobs with lower wages. When the 109th Congress again takes up the debate on mental health parity legislation, federal policymakers will be faced with the growing mental health and substance abuse treatment needs of rural Americans, which some argue are not being adequately addressed under our current patchwork system of regulations and programs for mental health care treatment (Gamm, Hutchison, Dabney, & Dorsey, 2003).

When the Mental Health Parity Act was enacted in 1996, Congress intended to address disparities in treatment of mental illness by establishing new federal standards for mental health coverage offered under most employer sponsored group health plans (U.S. General Accounting Office, 2000). However, the MHPA applied only to employer sponsored plans of 50 or more employees that fall under the umbrella of the Employee Retirement Income Security Act (ERISA). ERISA's complex provisions apply to employer sponsored or funded health insurance plans, and for that reason many of the insurance plans that might be available in a rural or frontier environment fall outside of ERISA's reach. As a result the provisions of MHPA do not apply to the millions of working-age Americans who live in rural areas and work for small employers (defined as less than 50 employees) or who are insured under a plan not covered by ERISA. For example the MHPA excludes individual insurance, nongroup plans, employer sponsored plans with 50 or fewer employees, and plans that experience an increase in claims costs (or the increased costs across an entire group plan) of one percent (U.S. General Accounting Office, 2000). Many of the health insurance plans available to those living in rural areas fall within these exclusions because rural employers tend to be smaller and are more likely not to offer group health coverage (Coburn, Kilbreth, Long, & Marquis, 1998). Even if they do offer employee benefit plans, individual claims costs are more likely to impact the group. Because of the MHPA's limited applicability, a significant percentage of rural workers were likely not helped by this initial and brief experiment expanding insurance coverage for mental diseases.

Rural workers, in general, have greater difficulty finding employer sponsored insurance because of smaller firm size and lower wages (Coburn, Kilbreth, Long & Marquis, 1998). Other research has shown that there are fewer firms offering health insurance in rural areas and employee participation rates are also lower. Consequently, many rural workers living just above poverty levels may be uninsured. Lack of health insurance creates significant problems for persons with mental illness who may need treatment in order to maintain ability to participate in work or other activities (National Council on Disability, 2002). Little is known about the individual effects of specific mental illnesses or the particular effects that rural regions may have in contributing to decreased work, absence of health insurance, or reduced wages for rural women suffering from mental illness. The focus of this research is on the specific effects of mental illness in contributing to unemployment, as well as its effects in contributing to lack of health insurance and lower wages.

RESEARCH OBJECTIVE

This research examines whether rural women with mental illness experience increased disadvantage in relation to reduced work activity in comparison with other women with chronic illnesses. This research also examines the probability that women with mental illness who manage to work will be unable to access health insurance and will have reduced wages in relation to other women with chronic illnesses or disabilities.

BACKGROUND AND SIGNIFICANCE

Rural America brings difficult challenges for anyone living there, but for rural working-age women it may be particularly difficult. Women living in rural America comprise 52% of the rural population and 30 percent of all women in the United States (Bergland, 1988). Yet, rural women are as diverse as the cultures, tribes, sects, regions, counties, and towns in which they live. Rural African-American women living in the deep South are very different from rural women in Nebraska, Arizona, or Alaska. However, all rural women, no matter where they live face similar, demanding economic challenges and, in fact, are more likely to be poorer than rural Caucasian males (American Psychological Association [APA], 1999; Hauenstein & Boyd, 1994). Higher rural poverty rates and fewer rural health care providers combine to increase the prevalence of chronic diseases and morbidity for those living in rural America. Demographically, women living in rural areas are less likely to have attended college, and more likely to live at or near the poverty level. On September 10, 2001, the Department of Health and Human Services and the National Center for Health Statistics (NCHS) released a report showing that rural residents lag behind suburban and urban residents in nearly all health status indicators (National Center for Health Statistics, 2001). Perhaps most significant of these health status indicators are statistics indicating that more rural women suffer from chronic illnesses than do their urban or suburban counterparts (APA, 1999). Some research indicates that prevalence of mental illness in rural areas is similar to nonrural areas, yet available and/or appropriate treatment is either nonexistent or more difficult to find in rural areas (National Institute of Mental Health [NIMH], 2001).

While prevalence rates of mental health disorders in the rural female population vary, in general it is agreed that rates of mental health disorders are as high in rural and frontier areas as in urban areas (APA, 1999; Wagenfeld, Murray, Mohatt, & DeBruyn, 1994). At least one other study has found evidence that rates of depression for rural women are as high as 40% in some areas (Hauenstein & Bashore, 2002). This compares to depression rates of 13–20 percent of women in urban areas. Suicide rates in many rural areas are higher than in urban areas. Recent testimony before Congress cited statistics showing that suicide rates in some rural areas (particularly the rural West) were twice as high as in the rest of the nation (Thomas, 2001). Moreover, the rate of serious mental illness in the rural population age 50 years old or older is 9.4 percent, significantly higher than for metro and urbanized areas (Substance Abuse and Mental Health Service Administration [SAMHSA], 2001).

Rural women with chronic mental illnesses and impairments may be particularly disadvantaged in relation to their urban counterparts because of higher poverty rates, head-of-household status, poorer maternal health, and higher prevalence of chronic illnesses (APA, 1999). Community support structures and appropriate treatment options are scarcer in most rural regions of the country (Gamm, Tai-Seale, & Stone, 2002).

It is well established that health insurance is an important determinant of access to health care services, including mental health treatment (Bolin & Gamm, 2003; Taylor, Cohen, & Machlin, 2001; Weinick, Zuvekas, & Drilea, 1997). As a result rural women, even if they do work, are likely to be disadvantaged in their ability to access treatment because of the fact that rural employers tend to be smaller, group health plans may not be offered, and work tends to be more scarce or sporadic. Therefore, rural women may find it more difficult to find or pay for any kind of mental health insurance (APA, 1999). Inability to find health insurance coverage is worse for African American and Hispanic women, both of whom are more likely than Whites to be uninsured (Bolin & Gamm, 2003; Hargraves, 2002; Mills, 2002).

Overall, African American and Hispanic women are more likely than White women to suffer racial or ethnic discrimination, have lower income levels, and work at low-status and/or high-stress jobs. Additional stress factors for these vulnerable groups include unemployment, poor health, larger family size, marital problems, and single parenthood (McGrath, Keita, Strickland, & Russo, 1990).

Unfortunately, adequate mental health care may be more difficult to find in rural areas. Sixty percent of rural areas are mental health professional shortage areas (APA, 1999). As a result, rural women suffering from mental illness who might have the ability to pay for treatment may find that a general practitioner must meet their mental health care needs, or that they must travel many miles for specialized care.

Often, in rural areas it is primarily only those in dire need or those in a psychiatric crisis, who receive in-patient treatment. Rates of incarceration for acute mental crises are higher in rural areas than in urban areas. Without preventive care or adequate mental health facilities, jails and prisons become treatment centers by default (National Council on Disability, 2002). Inmates in jails and prisons rarely receive optimum mental health treatment or community support for successful re-entry into the community. Finding cost-effective solutions to the difficulty of providing mental health care for the rural (primarily elderly) population, and preventing comorbidity, disability, and other consequences of mental illness is a significant national policy need (NIMH, 2001).

DATA, STUDY DESIGN, AND METHODS

Data

The data for this study comes from the combined 1994 and 1995 National Health Interview Surveys (NHIS-D) and their respective disability supplements. The 1994 and 1995 NHIS consists of a core survey, individual person record, and several supplements, including an insurance supplement, family resources supplement, and disability supplement, which were included in the data analyses. The 1994 and 1995 NHIS-D surveys were combined to obtain a sample of working-age women N = 21,970. Of these, 4,979 reside in rural areas. Included are 2,589 Hispanics, 3,456 Black non-Hispanics, and 15,175 White non-Hispanics. The sample consists of 15,963 women with a chronic physical condition; 2,575 with a mental condition, and 1,118 women with both mental and physical conditions. The NHIS-D used a complex survey design with sample population weights, clusters, and stratification. Because of the survey design, Stata's survey estimation program was used for simple two-way comparisons and survey analysis. However, due to small cell counts within certain clusters in the 1994 data set, the standard errors for survey estimation were not relied upon. Instead, comparisons between the standard errors in an ordinary probit and survey probit were made and compared to evaluate significance levels.

Study Design

This study was designed to answer three important research questions:

(1)   What are the differences in employment between rural and nonrural women with chronic mental and physical illnesses, across rural regions and by mental illness?

(2)   What are the differences in insurance status between rural and nonrural women with chronic mental and physical illnesses?

(3)   What are the differences in hourly earnings for rural women with mental illness, compared with nonrural women?

The research questions and hypotheses in this study are as follows:

H1:   Working-age women with mental illnesses living in rural areas are more likely not to work than working-age urban women with mental illnesses.

H2:   Working-age women with mental illnesses living in rural areas are more likely to be uninsured than working-age women with mental illness living in urban areas.

H3:   Working-age rural women with mental illnesses are more likely to earn less than working-age nonrural women with mental illnesses.

Analytical Methods

Descriptive statistics were first calculated to obtain demographic and illness-specific differences accounting for race, ethnicity, age, and rural region. This study then employs multivariate, single-stage and two-stage probit estimation techniques to model the likelihood of work activity, health insurance status, and hourly wages of women in the sample. Single-stage probit was utilized to predict the probability of any work and full-time work for women with mental illness. Two-stage probit was employed to estimate the likelihood of employer-sponsored insurance and the two-stage Heckman regression estimation to estimate the effect of mental illness on hourly wages. The multivariate model used to answer the research questions and test the hypotheses in this study is used to first estimate the effects of specific mental conditions and other individual level variables on the probability of working.

The probit probability distribution function of $Y = 1$ is expressed as:

$$Pr\ (Y_i^* = 1) = Pr\ (Z_i > 0) = 1 - F(Z_i > 0)(\alpha + \beta X_i + \varepsilon)$$

where $F\ (Z_i)$ is the cumulative density function of the standard normal distribution evaluated at Z_i, and $Z_i = \alpha + \beta X_i$ represents all of the individual parameters in the model and their individual coefficients. Model vectors are designated as follows:

Y = the outcome or dependent variable of interest. For Hypothesis 1 the DV is "**any work**" or "**full-time work**." For Hypothesis 2 the dependant variable in stage-2 is "**employer-sponsored insurance**." For Hypothesis 3, the dependent variable in stage-2 is "**log hourly wages**."

Z = a vector of individual predictors, including mental health condition, rural region, age, sex, education, children, marital status, race/ethnicity, and spouse's insurance and work status.

i = indexes the individual.

Because there may be differences in the effects of specific types of mental conditions, insurance status is evaluated using specific mental illness diagnoses as individual predictors. Significance testing was carried out using Z-statistics for the descriptive statistics; while Wald chi-square tests were used for the probit models.

PRINCIPAL FINDINGS

Descriptive Statistics: Rural women with *mental illness* are more likely to be unemployed than nonrural women with mental illness, 64 percent unemployed compared with 59 percent unemployed (p < .05). Rural women with mental illness are also more likely *not* to be working than either rural or nonrural females with a chronic *physical illness* (p < .05) (Table 6.1). In contrast, both rural and nonrural females who are healthy are significantly more likely to work full time. For both groups, 58 percent work full time. Rural females with mental illness are far less likely to work full time than nonrural women with mental illness, 24 percent versus 29 percent (p < .05). Nationally, rural females with mental illness are more likely to be on Medicare (28 percent) or Medicaid (46 percent) than their nonrural counterparts (p < .05).

Rural women with mental illness are significantly less likely to be the policy holder in an employer sponsored plan, 18 percent

TABLE 6.1 Employment and Insurance Status of Females with Mental and Physical Conditions by Rural and Nonrural Status (United States, 1994–1995 Population, Ages 25–64)

	Rural Females			Nonrural Females		
	Healthy	Mental	Physical	Healthy	Mental	Physical
Not Working	27%	64%	52%	27%	59%	46%
Working Part Time	17%	12%	14%	15%	12%	13%
Working Full Time	58%	24%	34%	58%	29%	41%
Uninsured	40%	13%	16%	36%	20%	13%
Policy Holder	42%	18%	32%	44%	23%	40%
Spouse Insured	56%	29%	46%	54%	30%	47%
Medicare	7%	28%	11%	5%	13%	7%
Medicaid	4%	46%	18%	5%	29%	14%
Other Public Insurance	2%	2%	1%	5%	4%	1%

Source: Author's computations from the 1994–1995 NHIS-D Surveys

compared with 23 percent for nonrural women (p < .05). Rural women with either a chronic mental or physical illness are much less likely to be the named insured on an employer-sponsored policy. There were no significant differences in percentages of those who were insured through their spouse between rural and nonrural women with a chronic mental or physical illness.

EMPLOYMENT RATES FOR SPECIFIC MENTAL ILLNESSES BY RURAL AND NONRURAL STATUS

The majority of rural women with mental illness do not work at all. However, employment rates vary by type of mental illness (Table 6.2). Rural women with schizophrenia or paranoia have an extremely high unemployment rate, 95 percent compared with 82 percent for nonrural women; followed by an 87 percent rural unemployment rate for women with a personality disorder, compared with 70 percent unemployment rate for nonrural women with a personality disorder.

Rural women with bipolar disorder have an 81 percent unemployment rate compared with 66 percent for nonrural women; followed by a 72 percent unemployment rate for depression, compared with 65 percent for nonrural, and a 56 percent unemployment rate for rural women with addiction disorders compared with 58 percent

TABLE 6.2   Employment Rates by Rural or Nonrural Status and Type of Mental Condition (United States, 1994–1995, Ages 25–64)

	Rural Females			Nonrural Females		
	Not Working	Part time	Full time	Not Working	Part time	Full time
Bipolar Disorder	81%	5%	14%	66%	12%	23%
Frequently Depressed	72%	10%	18%	65%	12%	24%
Schizophrenia/ Paranoia	95%	0.3%	5%	82%	9%	8%
Personality Disorder	87%	7%	6%	70%	10%	20%
Addiction Disorder	56%	12%	32%	58%	14%	28%

Source : Author's computations from the 1994–1995 NHIS-D Surveys

TABLE 6.3 Employment Rates of Rural Females with Mental Conditions by Region and Rural Status (United States, 1994–1995, Ages 25–64)

	Rural females with any mental illness			
	No Work	Part Time	Full Time	Uninsured
Rural North East	54%	18%	28%	27%
Rural Midwest	64%	7%	29%	11%
Rural South	86%	5%	9%	19%
Rural West	79%	8%	13%	13%

Source: Author's computations from the 1994–1995 NHIS-D Surveys

for nonrural. These differences in percentage estimates are all significant at p < .05.

Employment Status of Females with Any Mental Illness by Rural Region

Table 6.3 shows significant differences in overall employment rates across rural regions for females with *any* kind of mental illness. For example, women with any kind of mental illness living in the rural South have an extremely high unemployment rate of 86 percent and appear to be particularly disadvantaged in terms of finding suitable work. The rural South is followed by the rural West with an unemployment rate of 79 percent, followed by the rural Midwest at 64 percent, and the rural Northeast at 54 percent. These estimates are all significant at p < .05.

Uninsured Rates by Type of Mental Illness, Race/Ethnicity, and Rural Region

Depending upon the state of residence, rural women with mental illness may not qualify for SSI and Medicaid, despite sporadic employment and living near poverty. Such women tend to fall between the cracks in terms of ability to find or maintain jobs offering employer-sponsored health insurance, yet may not qualify for public insurance such as Medicaid. Table 6.4 provides estimates of rural women who are *completely uninsured* (no employer-sponsored or

TABLE 6.4 Uninsured Rates by Race/Ethnicity and by Type of Mental Illness According to Rural/Nonrural Status (United States, 1995 Population, Ages 25–64)

	White Non-Hispanic		Black Non-Hispanic		Hispanic		Other Non-Hispanic	
	Rural	Non-rural	Rural	Non-rural	Rural	Non-rural	Rural	Non-rural
Any Mental Disorder	17%	17%	15%	20%	38%	25%	6%	9%
Addiction Disorder	25%	17%	10%	19%	77%	18%	0%	0%
Personality Disorder	8%	17%	0%	24%	51%	35%	0%	14%
Depression	17%	17%	15%	20%	36%	25%	6%	8%
Schizophrenia/ Paranoia	12%	16%	12%	6%	20%	30%	0%	30%

Source: Author's computations from the 1994–1995 NHIS-D Surveys

public insurance), by type of mental illness and by race or ethnicity. It should be noted that low cell counts for bipolar disorder prevented comparisons by both race/ethnicity and rural/nonrural status, that the combined 1994–1995 NHIS Disability data sets did not have observations of rural "Other non-Hispanic" available for analysis. The "Other non-Hispanic" race and ethnicity category comprises Asians, Pacific Islanders, American Indians, and Eskimos.

In Table 6.4 we see that rural Hispanic females have the highest uninsured rates across all mental disease classifications. For any mental illness, rural Hispanic females have a 38 percent uninsured rate, compared with 25 percent for nonrural females ($p < .05$). Moreover, Hispanic females with mental disease experience significantly higher uninsured rates than either White non-Hispanic or Black non-Hispanic females in any category of mental disease.

MULTIVARIATE RESULTS

Probability of Work for Women with Mental Illness

The results of multivariate probit analyses support the hypothesis that working age women with mental illnesses living in rural areas are more likely not to work than working-age nonrural women with mental illnesses. All three models are estimated using the entire sample (rural and nonrural) of working-age women with one or more chronic disease or impairment. Our analyses are directed to the effects of mental illness reported by women in the sample. The impact of specific mental illnesses on any work or full-time work is (with the exception of addiction disorder) negative and significant. In addition, women living in rural regions in the South and West have an additional negative likelihood of not finding any work (p < .05).

In Table 6.5 we observe the coefficients of specific mental disorders and rural region (along with other important work predictors)

TABLE 6.5 Single-Equation Models of Employment Status for Females with Mental Conditions

	Any Work		Full-Time Work	
	Coefficients	Marginal Effects	Coefficients	Marginal Effects
Bipolar disorder	−0.23*	−0.09	−0.23*	−0.08
Personality disorder	−0.23*	−0.09	−0.18*	−0.07
Addiction disorder	−0.14	−0.06	−0.27**	−0.10
Schizophrenia/ paranoia	−0.79***	−0.30	−0.76***	−0.25
Depression disorder	−0.52***	−0.20	−0.48***	−0.18
Rural Northeast	−0.08	−0.03	−0.13*	−0.05
Rural South	−0.09**	−0.04	−0.04	−0.02
Rural West	−0.14**	−0.06	−0.21***	−0.08
Black non-Hispanic	−0.20***	−0.08	−0.07**	−0.03
Other non-Hispanic	−0.05	−0.02	0.08	0.03
Hispanic	−0.16***	−0.06	−0.08**	−0.03
Constant	0.11**		−0.20***	

N = 16,822
Prob Y = 1 at means of X's
*P < .1
**P < .05
***P < .01

Full tables containing all statistical coefficients available upon request from jbolin@srph. tamushsc.edu.

on the work activity of all women in the sample who reported a chronic mental or physical disorder. The probability of "any work" (1–90 hrs/week) for females with bipolar disorder and personality disorder was negative with marginal effects (the specific effects of an indicator in changing the probability from 0 to 1) for both at −0.09 (p < .004). The marginal effect of schizophrenia was large and negative at −0.30 percent (p < .000); and nearly as large for depression at −0.20 percent (p < .000).

Women in the sample who live in the rural South were also less likely to work than women living in the rural Midwest (−0.04 percent) (p < .000). Likewise women living in the rural Northeast and rural West are less likely to find work than rural women living in the Midwest. The marginal effects of *full-time employment* were larger, with the biggest effect seen in the rural West (−0.08 percent) followed by the rural Northeast (−0.05), and rural South (−0.02). Hispanic, Black non-Hispanics, and other non-White racial/ethnic groups have an additional reduced probability of part-time or full-time employment. For example, the marginal effects for full time work are −0.03 percent for Hispanics and Black non-Hispanics (p < .05).

TWO-STAGE MULTIVARIATE PROBIT ANALYSES

Likelihood of Having Employer Sponsored Insurance, if Working

Access to employer sponsored health insurance varies according to type of mental disease, rural region, and whether a given woman works full time or at all (Table 6.6). Women with schizophrenia or paranoia have a high probability of being unemployed, and even if they do happen to work full time (or > 35 hrs per week, thus qualifying for insurance), they are more likely *not* to be offered health insurance. The marginal effects for women with schizophrenia and paranoia shown in Table 6.6 are −.22 percent (p < .05). Women suffering from depression are less likely to access health insurance through their employer if they work (−.14 percent). Working women living in the rural West and rural South with a chronic mental illness have an additional negative likelihood of having health insurance at −.15 and −.04 respectively (p < .001).

TABLE 6.6 Two-Equation Probit Models Predicting Employer Insurance for Working Females by Conditions

	Working At All			Employer Insurance Working Full Time		
	Any Work	Employer Insurance	Marginal Effects	Full time	Employer Insurance	Marginal Effects
Bipolar disorder	−0.20***	−0.11	−0.04	−0.12*	0.08	0.03
Personality disorder	−0.22***	0.06	0.02	−0.26***	−0.08	−0.03
Addiction disorder	0.01	−0.09	−0.04	−0.06	−0.12	−0.05
Schizophrenia/ paranoia	−0.78***	−0.67***	−0.22	−0.93***	−0.63***	−0.21
Depression disorder	−0.56***	−0.39***	−0.14	−0.55***	−0.37***	−0.13
Rural Northeast	−0.13**	−0.13	−0.05	−0.23***	−0.18*	−0.07
Rural South	−0.13***	−0.11**	−0.04	−0.10***	−0.15***	−0.06
Rural West	−0.09**	−0.41***	−0.15	−0.21***	−0.40** *	−0.14
Black non-Hispanic	−0.24***	−0.08*	−0.03	−0.11***	−0.10**	−0.04
Other non-Hispanic	−0.23***	−0.17**	−0.06	−0.07	−0.20***	−0.07
Hispanic	−0.14***	−0.08**	−0.03	−0.06**	−0.05	−0.02
Constant	−0.09***	−0.18		−0.40***	−0.27	
N = 21,970						
Rho		0.82			0.60	
Chi^2		***			***	
Prob Y = 1 at the means of X's			0.28			0.37

* p < .10
** p < .05
*** p < .01

Full tables containing all statistical coefficients available upon request from jbolin@srph.tamushsc.edu

The Effect of Mental Illness on Hourly Wages

With the exception of addiction disorders, the effect of having a mental illness on a woman's wage rate is negative. However, only bipolar disorder, schizophrenia/paranoia and depression were significant at .05 or higher. In Table 6.7 the two-stage Heckman estimates of the effects of mental illnesses on hourly wage rates (using log hourly wages) are set out for *any work* and *full-time* work. These estimates were performed using the Stata8® survey estimation statistical package.

For women performing *any work*, bipolar disorder has a significant and negative effect on wages (−32 percent) (p < .05). For women performing *full-time* work, bipolar disorder, schizophrenia, and depression had a large and significant negative effect on wages, −40.6 for schizophrenia, −6.8 percent for depression, and −16.8 for bipolar disorder (p < .05). Women who live in the rural South have an additional likelihood of reduced wages (compared with other women with chronic illnesses) for both any work and full-time work. Interestingly, women in the rural West who manage to work despite their mental illness have a +31.4 percent likelihood of higher hourly wages for any work compared with rural women from the Midwest, and a +33.7 percent likelihood of higher hourly wages for full-time work compared with rural women from the Midwest. The reason for this difference is not apparent.

DISCUSSION

The results of this research demonstrate that women with chronic mental illnesses living in rural areas have reduced work and lower wages compared with their urban counterparts. Rural women, especially minorities, are also more likely *not* to have job-based health insurance, even if working. Moreover, women living in the rural South and rural West face an even greater disadvantage in accessing health insurance than women in the rural Midwest. These disparities are even more significant for rural African American and Hispanic women. Disparity in ability to access insurance is important for rural women in need of mental health services and other health care, because a lack of health insurance coverage is inextricably linked

TABLE 6.7 Two-Equation Models of Log Hourly Wage for Females with Mental Conditions Using Survey Estimation Methods

	Effect of Mental Conditions on Log Hourly Wage					
	Any Work	Change in Wage	Percent Change	Full-time Work	Change in Wage	Percent Change
Bipolar disorder	−0.19***	−0.32***	−28	−0.14*	−0.18*	−17.0
Personality disorder	−0.24***	−0.03	−2.5	−0.26***	0.13	−13.6
Addiction disorder	−0.02	0.14	15	−0.08	0.11	−12.0
Schizophrenia/ paranoia	−0.76***	−0.11	−11	−0.83***	−0.52***	−40.6
Depression disorder	−0.55***	−0.06	−5.9	−0.56***	−0.07*	−6.8
Rural Northeast	−0.10*	−0.06	−5.7	−0.17***	−0.13	−12.0
Rural South	−0.14***	−0.18***	−17	−0.09***	−0.26***	−23.0
Rural West	−0.15***	0.27***	31.4	−0.23***	0.29**	−33.8
Black non-Hispanic	−0.22***	−0.11***	−10.1	−0.10***	−0.09***	−8.5
Other non-Hispanic	−0.18***	−0.13**	−11.8	−0.01	−0.12**	−11.0
Hispanic	−0.15***	−0.09*	−8.3	−0.08**	−0.10**	−9.4
Constant	−0.01	3.14***		−0.29***	3.20***	
N = 21,943						
Rho	−0.05			−0.02		
Wald Chi2	431.4			467.7		
Significance	***			***		

* $p < .1$
** $p < .05$
*** $p < .01$

Full tables containing all statistical coefficients available upon request from jbolin@srph.tamushsc.edu

to preventive care, faster health decline, and earlier death (Bolin & Gamm, 2003; Institute of Medicine, 2002; Strickland & Strickland, 1996).

One of the biggest challenges facing the 109th Congress will be addressing the mental health care needs of vulnerable groups within the rural population, such as minorities and women. Our present system of linking mental health insurance coverage to employers with 50 or more employees who happen to offer group health insurance effectively precludes many working-age rural women with chronic mental illnesses from finding adequate or appropriate mental health treatment. The unique conditions and environment of nearly every rural region in America, the most important of which are poverty and short supply of mental health providers, place those who are most needy at the greatest risk of receiving no or inadequate treatment for their mental illnesses. Despite attempts by Congress to address disparity in mental health coverage through *The Mental Health Parity Act*, the Act does little to address the needs of rural women with mental illness, given their reduced rates of employment and isolated existence. If Congress is to adequately address the mental health needs of rural women, it ought to carefully craft mental health parity legislation that improves access to rural mental health treatment services, increases the number of rural mental health specialists, including psychologists and psychiatrists, and enable small communities to provide community support services and education services for women with mental illness who may also be victims of abuse, crime, and/or extreme poverty.

REFERENCES

American Psychological Association (1999). *The Behavioral Health Care Needs of Rural Women*. Retrieved October 2002, from http://www.apa.org/rural/ruralwomen.pdf

Bergland, B. (1988). Rural mental health: Report of the National Action Commission on the Mental Health of Rural Americans. *Journal of Rural Community Psychology, 9*(2), 29–39.

Bolin, J., & Gamm, L. (2003). Access to Quality Health Services in Rural Areas—Insurance: A Literature Review. In L. D. Gamm, L. L. Hutchison, B. J. Dabney, & A. M. Dorsey (Eds.), *Rural Healthy People 2010: A companion document to Healthy People 2010* (Vol. 2). College Station, TX: The Texas A&M University System Health Science Center, School of Rural Public Health, Southwest Rural Health Research Center.

Center for Medicare and Medicaid Services (2003, June). 45 CFR Part 146; Amendment to the Interim Final Regulation for Mental Health Services; *Federal Register, 68*(124).

Coburn, A. F., Kilbreth, E. H., Long, S. H., & Marquis, M. S. (1998). Urban-rural differences in employer-based health insurance coverage of workers, *Medical Care Research and Review, 55*(4), 484–496.

Department of Labor, Employee Benefits Security Administration (2003). Mental Health Parity, 29 CFR, Part 2590; *Federal Register 68*(71), 18048–18050.

Gamm, L. D., Tai-Seale, M., & Stone, S. (2002). White Paper: Meeting the Mental Health Needs of People Living in Rural Areas. Center for Mental Health Services, Substance Abuse and Mental Health Services Administration. Washington, D.C.

Gamm, L. D., Hutchison, L. L., Dabney, B. J., & Dorsey, A. M. (Eds.). (2003). *Rural Healthy People 2010: A Companion Document to Healthy People 2010* (Vols. 1–2). College Station, TX: The Texas A&M University System Health Science Center, School of Rural Public Health, Southwest Rural Health Research Center.

Hargraves, J. L. (2002). The insurance gap and minority health care, 1997–2001. Center for Studying Health Systems Change, Tracking Report No. 2:1–4.

Hauenstein, E. J., & Bashore, R. T. (2002, October). Press Release. University of Virginia, School of Nursing.

Hauenstein, E. J., & Boyd, M. R., (1994). Depressive symptoms in young women of the Piedmont: Prevalence in rural women. *Women and Health, 21*(2/3), 105–123.

Institute of Medicine (2002). *Care without coverage: Too little, too late.* Washington, DC: National Academy of Sciences.

McGrath, E., Keita, G. P., Strickland, B. R., & Russo, N. (Eds.). (1990). *Women and depression: Risk factors and treatment issues.* Washington, DC: American Psychological Association.

Mills, R. J. (2002, September). Health Insurance Coverage: 2001. U.S. Census Bureau, Washington, D.C. Retrieved July 10, 2003, from http://www.census.gov/prod/2002pubs/p60-220.pdf

National Center for Health Statistics (2001). *Health, United States, 2001 with urban and rural health chartbook.* Hyattsville, MD: Author.

National Council on Disability (2002, September). The Well Being of Our Nation: An Inter-Generational Vision of Effective Mental Health Services and Supports. Retrieved October 7, 2002, from http://www.ncd.gov/newsroom/publications/2002/mentalhealth.htm

National Institute of Mental Health (2001). Report of the Workgroup on Mental Disorders Prevention; Executive Summary. Retrieved October 4, 2004, from http://journals.apa.org/prevention/volume4/pre0040017a.html

Strickland, J., & Strickland, D. L. (1996). Barriers to preventive health services for minority households in the rural south. *Journal of Rural Health, 12*(3), 206–217.

Substance Abuse and Mental Health Services Administration (2001). 2001 National Household Survey on Drug Abuse, Mental Health Tables.Retrieved October 14, 2002, from http://www.oas.samhsa.gov/nhsda/2k1nhsda/vol1/toc.htm

Taylor, A., Cohen, J., & Machlin, S. (2001). Being uninsured in 1996 compared to 1987: How has the experience of the uninsured changed over time? *Health Services Research, 36*(6), 16–31.

Thomas, C. (2001, May). Press Release: Thomas Drafts Rural Health Legislation Retrieved October 14, 2002, from http://thomas.senate.gov/html/pr362.html

U.S. General Accounting Office (2000). Mental health parity act: Employers' mental health benefits remain limited despite new federal standards, GAO/ T-HEHS-00-113.

Wagenfeld, M. O., Murray, J. D., Mohatt, D. F., & DeBruyn, J. C. (1994). *Mental health and rural America: 1980–1993.* An Overview and Annotated Bibliography (NIH Publication No. 94-3500). Washington, DC: Office of Rural Health Policy.

Weinick, R., Zuvekas, S., & Drilea, S. (1997). Access to health care:Sources and barriers, 1996 (MEPS Research Findings No. 3, AHCPR Pub. No. 98-001). Rockville, MD: Agency for Health Care Policy and Research.

Chapter 7

Mental Health Care Utilization and Expenditures Among Rural Women

Judith Shinogle

INTRODUCTION

The burden of mental illness on the health of the United States population is a growing area of concern highlighted in the U.S. Surgeon General's Report on Mental Health (U.S. Department of Health and Human Services, 1999). Data from the Global Burden of Disease study indicate that mental health is second only to cardiovascular conditions in the burden of disease in established market economies such as the United States (Murray & Lopez, 1996). About 15 percent of the U.S. adult population use services from the mental health services sector in a year (U.S. Department of Health and Human Services, 1999). Evidence suggests that the prevalence of mental illness and substance abuse is similar in rural and urban adults (Kessler et al., 1994). While this equal prevalence may exist, it is well established that rural areas have fewer mental health services than urban areas (Ricketts, 1999). Besides the lack of services for mental health and substance abuse in rural areas, distance from a service provider and travel time may add to the difficulty of obtaining treatment.

Another concern for providing mental health services in rural areas is the stigma associated with mental illness. Studies have shown that depressed rural residents are more likely to negatively label people who sought professional help for treatment (Rost, Smith, & Taylor, 1993), and the lack of anonymity in small towns and rural environments may exacerbate the influence of this stigma.

For females in rural areas, mental health utilization is of particular interest since the incidence of mental health problems is higher in females (U.S. Department of Health and Human Services, 1999). While previous studies have examined mental health utilization in rural areas, only a few have examined expenditures and none have focused specifically on females. The analysis presented in this chapter attempts to fill this void by examining factors associated with mental health utilization and expenditures for females. In addition, this chapter will focus on rural African American women.

Research has consistently shown that rural patients are less likely to have access to mental health specialists and thus generally have fewer specialty visits. One study found that depressed rural patients have fewer mental health specialty visits and slightly more inpatient visits (Rost, Zhang, Fortney, Smith, & Smith, 1998). Another study found that patients receiving treatment from a managed care organization in a more rural community received more mental health services from primary care physicians and had more inpatient utilization than their counterparts receiving care from a managed care organization in a less rural setting (Yuen, Gerdes, & Gonzales, 1996).

Few studies examine minority mental health and/or substance abuse treatment utilization. Thomas and Snowden (2001) used the 1987 National Medical Expenditure Survey to study mental health treatment of minorities. They found that minorities with private health insurance use fewer mental health services than Whites with private health insurance. In addition, their study found minorities with private health insurance use fewer mental health services than minorities with public health insurance (Thomas & Snowden, 2001).

While this study provides information on minority mental health treatment, the study did not consider the impact of rural/urban residency. Although the study did not find any significant effect of sex on mental health utilization, the regression model developed in the study did control for sex. Since females have a higher incidence of mental disorders, a separate model for females may provide more information on the effects of sex on utilization as well as expenditures.

One study has examined sex difference in utilization of outpatient mental health services. Rhodes, Goering, To, and Williams (2002) found that females had higher odds of outpatient mental health use, even after adjustments for disease type and age in a Canadian population. They did not find any difference in volume (i.e., number of visits), only in likelihood of use. This study highlights the fact that the female population may be more likely to use mental health services, but the researchers did not explore utilization of other mental health services (such as prescription drugs), nor did their study examine mental health expenditures. In addition, the study by Rhodes and colleagues (2002) did not specifically investigate rural females. Finally, the study was in a different health care system (Canada) and thus this study may not be generalizable to the U.S. population.

While previous studies have examined differences in utilization between rural and urban populations, few have examined differences in expenditures or the amounts paid out of pocket for mental health and substance abuse treatment. Ringel and Sturm (2001) examined mental health expenditures using a nationally representative data set. They found that females may have lower mean out-of-pocket expenditures for mental health services. However, when analyzed according to mean share of income, or the percentage of people with a significant burden (defined as paying for 50 percent or more of total mental health costs out of pocket), females always pay a higher percentage of available income than males. What is particularly noteworthy is that this higher out-of-pocket burden did not exist for the minority population. The effect on rural females or rural minority females is not clear from this study.

The goal of this chapter is to provide a descriptive picture of rural female mental health and substance abuse treatment utilization and expenditures using a nationally representative sample. The emphasis of the analysis is to describe differences in utilization and expenditures for rural minority women. Rural minority women may be at higher risk for poor outcomes due to a lack of adequate internal (education) and external (health insurance) resources.

The following research questions were examined with a focus on differences between urban and rural women: 1) Which factors are associated with women receiving mental health and/or substance abuse treatment? 2) Among those women who received treatment, what is the likelihood that they received services in an office-based setting?[1] and 3) Among those women who received treatment, what is the likelihood that they received prescription drugs as part of their mental health and/or substance abuse treatment? In addition, the study compared urban and rural women on the total amount of mental health and substance abuse treatment expenditures, the amount paid out of pocket, and the percentage of personal income that was spent out of pocket on mental health and substance abuse treatment. Finally, the study examined all of these questions with a special emphasis on how rural African American women differed from White rural and urban women.

METHODS

Data

The data utilized in the present study was obtained from the 1996 and 1997 Medical Expenditure Panel Survey (MEPS). The MEPS is a nationally representative sample of the U.S. noninstitutionalized civilian population conducted by the Agency for Healthcare Research Quality (AHRQ). The MEPS provides data on health care services use, expenditures, and source of payment as well as data on the individual's economic, demographic, family, and other characteristics. MEPS provides detailed event[2] files that contain specific information regarding associated diagnoses for each event as well as expenditures and source of payment for each event. In order to identify mental health utilization, diagnosis codes were used to identify an event associated with mental health and/or substance abuse (MHSA) diagnosis.[3] Individuals were categorized as having a mental health utilization and/or substance abuse treatment if any of three condition codes associated with an event was a mental health and/or substance abuse code. The event files examined include inpatient, outpatient, emergency room, office-based visits, and prescription drugs. It excluded home health, other medical devices, and dental services. To obtain the two expenditure variables, the total expenditures and amount paid out of pocket for the mental health and/or substance abuse events were summed to a person-level variable.

All analyses were limited to females. In addition, since types of mental health disorders and substance abuse vary by age, the analyses were also limited to individuals age 18 and over. Finally, for some cases, independent variables (such as education level, rural status, etc.) were missing or coded as "respondent did not know" or "unknown." These observations were deleted from the data set. There may be concerns as to whether these variables are truly missing. Thus, it is suggested that other methods, such as imputation, may be used in the future to include all observations. With these exclusions, the remaining data for 1996 included unweighted observations of 8,338 individuals that, when weighted with survey sample weights, represent a national sample of 110,600,000 females, and for 1997 unweighted observations of 12,745 individuals that, when weighted with survey sample weights, represent a national sample of 102,300,000 females. For the analysis describing the percentage of out of pocket expenditures to income, those cases with missing or zero income were deleted, and thus, for this analysis, the sample has unweighted observations of 7,615 for 1996 and 10,862 for 1997.

Variable Definitions

For this analysis, rural was defined as residing in an area that is not a metropolitan statistical area (MSA). This measure would classify as "rural," females who live in areas adjacent to urban metropolitan areas. While this definition may dilute the truly rural population, for most national data sets this is the only definition available. Insurance coverage was defined by three mutually exclusive variables: any private health insurance (including private health insurance, employer- or union-sponsored health insurance, other private sources of health insurance, as well as CHAMPUS and Veterans Administration), public coverage only (Medicare, Medicaid, and/or other public health insurance), or uninsured all year. Health status was measured by two self-reported variables. In the MEPS survey respondents were asked to rate their general health and mental health on a five-point scale (poor, fair, good, very good, or excellent) in specific rounds of the survey. Fair or poor mental health status was coded as "1" if the female reported either of these measures during any round in the survey for that year. A fair or poor general health indicator was coded in the same manner. Females were defined as employed if their employment status was either employed on December 31st of the year, planning to return to work, working part of the year, or self-employed during the year. Finally, personal income included all forms of income for the person except sales income and income tax refunds.

Statistical Analyses

All statistical analyses were performed separately for each year. Since MEPS has a complex survey design, all analyses were performed using survey weights, primary sampling units, and strata as defined by the documentation and analyzed with Stata™ survey commands. To describe the data, a simple bivariate analysis was performed on important confounding variables comparing rural versus urban, using Chi-Square tests for categorical variables (marital status, poverty status, insurance coverage, race, region, educational attainment, employment status, general health status, and mental health status) and t-tests for continuous variables (age, income, and expenditures).

Several different main outcome variables were examined to study mental health and/or substance abuse treatment. The first was a dichotomous variable coded as "1" if the female had any mental health utilization during the year and "0" otherwise. To gain a better understanding of the type of services, additional variables were analyzed including the percentage of mental health utilizers who reported any use of prescription drugs, any office-based visits, any inpatient stays, any emergency room visits, and any outpatient visits for mental health and/or substance abuse treatment during the year. These variables were examined for rural-urban differences in these percentages. To examine the costs of mental health and substance abuse treatment services, the total mental health and substance abuse treatment expenditures and the amount of mental health and substance abuse treatment expenditures paid out of pocket were analyzed. In addition to measuring the financial burden of mental health expenditures, the percent of income spent on mental health and substance abuse treatment expenditures was also examined. All outcome variables were tested for rural-urban differences using chi-square tests for categorical variables (any mental health and/or substance abuse treatment, any use of prescription drugs, any office-based visits, any inpatient stays, any emergency room visits, and any outpatient visits) and t-tests for continuous variables (total expenditures, out of pocket expenditures, and percentage of income spent on out of pocket expenditures).

Finally, to control for possible confounders, a multiple logistic regression analysis was performed to examine factors associated with a person having any mental health and/or substance abuse treatment utilization. Again, to examine type of service utilized, two other dependent variables were analyzed using logistic regression: 1) any prescription drug use among those with any mental health utilization and 2) any office-based use among those with any mental health utilization. These services were chosen due to the higher percentage of females that reported utilizing these services and to increase the reliability of these estimates compared with other services where the outcome was rare.

To explore factors associated with total mental health expenditures and amount paid out of pocket, simple regression models as well as generalized linear models were utilized. Generalized linear models using a log link were employed due to the skewed nature of the expenditures data (Manning & Mullahy, 2001). The coefficients were of similar magnitude and sign to models using ordinary least squares, and thus the discussion will focus on the simple linear regression results.

To examine if there is a differential effect for being both rural and African American, in all of the multivariate models the associations of minority rural residents were tested to detect differences in the likelihood of outcomes studied through two interaction variables: 1) rural status multiplied by African American and 2) rural status multiplied by Hispanic non-African American. Because of the small cell size, and thus unreliable estimates with the Hispanic-rural interaction, the results section focuses the discussion on the African American-rural interaction. All models also included the following independent variables: marital status, age, age squared, indicators for poverty level, indicators for region, rural status, and race. Other independent variables included in the model are indicators for public health insurance only coverage, for being uninsured all year, for high school or greater education, for being employed, and for fair or poor mental health status. These variables were chosen because they are likely to be associated with occurrence of a mental disorder or with the likelihood of obtaining treatment for a mental disorder. The regression models include insurance status that may bias the coefficient estimates due to the inability to control for unobserved variables such as severity of illness, risk preferences, etc., that affect both the woman's choice of insurance as well MHSA treatment. Not controlling for these omitted variables could lead to biased estimates. This will be discussed further in the limitations section.

RESULTS

The results were similar in both 1996 and 1997. The bivariate analyses comparing the metropolitan statistical area (MSA) to non-MSA females are presented in Table 7.1. Rural women are more likely to be White (80 percent vs. 72 percent), married (58 percent vs. 54 percent), and slightly older (47 years old vs. 45 years old) than their urban counterparts.

Rural women are a vulnerable population in that they are more likely to have lower income. Approximately 20 percent (19 percent in 1996 and 18 percent in 1997) are in the 125–199 percent of poverty income level. Rural women are therefore at risk for lower access to health insurance because they may be ineligible for Medicaid and at the same time may not have access to private health insurance coverage. In addition, rural women are less educated than their urban counterparts; approximately 20 percent (in both years) have bachelor's or advanced degrees. This is a concern since education is a representation of investment in one's self and the creation of human capital. Moreover, investment in health and education is usually associated with increased ability to access the health care system and a greater ability to use medical treatments appropriately.

Finally, rural women are more likely than urban women to be uninsured all year (13 percent for rural vs. 10 percent for urban). This difference is important, especially in the examination of mental health and substance abuse treatment utilization and expenditures. Studies have shown that private health insurance often places stricter limits on the coverage for mental health and substance abuse

TABLE 7.1   Means of Variables in Analysis

	1996			1997		
	NonMSA	MSA	Total	NonMSA	MSA	Total
Poverty Level*						
< 100%	15.73%	13.27%	13.75%	16.25%	12.18%	12.98%
100 to 124%	7.15%	4.36%	4.91%	5.45%	4.56%	4.74%
125 to 199%	19.36%	14.15%	15.18%	17.93%	13.25%	14.17%
200 to 399%	34.31%	31.33%	31.91%	35.49%	31.33%	32.15%
> 400%	23.46%	36.88%	34.24%	24.88%	38.69%	35.96%
			p value < .001			p value < .001
Race*						
Hispanic	3.95%	10.51%	9.22%	4.03%	10.74%	9.41%
Black	9.20%	12.75%	12.05%	8.95%	13.00%	12.20%
Other	2.54%	4.49%	4.10%	2.13%	4.47%	4.01%
White	84.31%	72.26%	74.62%	84.88%	71.79%	74.37%
			p value < .001			p value < .001
Educational Attainment*						
No degree	22.38%	16.89%	17.96%	22.54%	16.54%	17.72%
High school or GED	57.45%	54.00%	54.68%	58.68%	54.12%	55.02%
Bachelor's	9.06%	15.59%	14.31%	8.28%	15.52%	14.09%
Advanced	11.11%	13.53%	13.05%	10.49%	13.82%	13.17%
			p value < .001			p value < .001
Insurance Coverage*						
Any private	71.86%	75.79%	75.02%	70.66%	75.25%	74.34%
Public only	14.58%	14.20%	14.27%	15.98%	14.74%	14.99%
Uninsured all year	13.56%	10.01%	10.71%	13.36%	10.00%	10.67%
			p value < .011			p value .002
Employed	63.83%	67.47%	66.75%	65.59%	68.30%	67.76%
			p value.040			p value.090
Married*	57.58%	53.86%	54.60%	58.52%	53.44%	54.45%
			p value < .001			p value < .001
Age*	46.53	45.15	45.42	46.87	45.34	45.64
			p value .040			p value .005

*p < .05
**p < .01
***p < .001

treatment than on coverage for general health (Salkever, Shinogle, & Goldman, 1999). Public health programs have fewer restrictions or the coverage for mental health and substance abuse treatment is equal to that for general health (see Center for Medicare and Medicaid Services website, http://www.cms.hhs.gov). This difference in generosity may influence the utilization as well as the total expenditures and amount paid out of pocket. On the other hand, the lack of insurance, i.e., higher percentage of uninsured in the rural female population may create a barrier to care that would decrease the ability of rural women to have access to the health care system.

These circumstances affecting rural females may place them at risk for poorer mental health status and decreased utilization of health services, yet this was found not to be the case in this analysis. Table 7.2 presents the rural-urban differences in mental health outcomes used in this study. As seen in the first row, there is no difference in self-reported poor or fair mental health status between rural and urban women (10 percent for rural and 9 percent for urban, p = .466), yet rural women do report significantly lower general health status than urban women (p = .023). In 1996, 23 percent of rural women reported fair to poor general health, while only 19 percent of urban women reported fair to poor health status. In 1997, a larger percentage of rural (26 percent) and urban (22 percent) women reported fair to poor health status, although the difference between rural and urban women remained approximately the same (p = .010).

No difference was found in the percentage of rural women who utilized any mental health services (11 percent in 1996 and 10 percent in 1997, p = .147, p = .888) when compared with urban women (approximately 10 percent in both years). This could be viewed positively as an indication that rural women who need mental health treatment are actually obtaining it. This analysis does not control for confounders, however, nor does it provide a causal analysis since the data is cross-sectional in nature and such a conclusion cannot be made. On the other hand, there are some women (both rural and urban) who rate their mental health as poor or fair, yet do not seek treatment in the traditional health care system. For rural women, 23 percent reported fair or poor mental health status, yet only 10 percent were receiving any mental health treatment. This may be due to underreporting of mental health treatment in the

TABLE 7.2   Health Status and Mental Health Care Utilization

	NonMSA	1996 MSA	Total	p-value	Non-MSA
Fair/poor mental health	10.07%	9.19%	9.37%	.466	10.87%
Fair/poor general health*	22.93%	19.23%	19.95%	.023	25.55%
Any mental health/ substance abuse utilization	10.94%	9.66%	9.91%	.145	10.47%
For those with any mental health/substance abuse utilization:					
Any MHSA prescription drug*	89.70%	82.80%	84.30%	.042	86.20%
Any MHSA office-based	53.88%	59.01%	57.89%	.260	55.40%
Any MHSA inpatient	3.88%	2.99%	3.18%	.618	6.64%
Any MHSA emergency room	2.07%	2.50%	2.41%	.755	2.16%
Any MHSA outpatient	5.68%	4.04%	4.40%	.447	1.78%
Mental health/substance abuse expenditures for those with any missing information					
Total expenditures	$969.62	$1,087.79	$1,062.15	.649	$1,593.71
Out of pocket expenditures**	$157.43	$306.47	$247.14	.003	$205.25
Fraction of out of pocket MH $ to income	0.009	0.014	0.014	.599	0.012
Income **	$16,821	$22,446	$19,839	.001	$17,412

* $p < .05$
** $p < .01$
*** $p < .001$

data, but also may be indicative of the unmet need occurring in mental health and substance abuse treatment for women.

To gain a better understanding of the type of mental health services women are utilizing, the type of services the women received was examined. This analysis was limited to those females with any mental health and/or substance abuse utilization. Table 7.2 provides the bivariate analysis comparing the rural-urban differences in the percentage of women who had any prescription drug treatment, office-based visits, inpatient days, emergency room visits, or outpatient visits during the year analyzed. A significantly higher percentage of rural women used prescription drugs compared with nonrural women in 1996 (p = .044) but this difference was not consistently significant across the two years studied. The results are similar to those of previous studies in that a higher percentage of the rural population used inpatient or emergency-room services when compared with the nonrural population, while a lower percentage used office-based visits. While none of these differences were consistently significant, they suggest that rural women are less likely to obtain mental health services in a nonacute care setting. This difference could be attributed to the lack of supply or demand for these types of services. Again, one must be cautious in the interpretation of these results in this simple bivariate analysis due to the potential presence of confounding factors. In addition, the effects of selection bias and unobserved heterogeneity in mental health severity were not controlled in this analysis. Furthermore, the small numbers in some of the cells make any national estimates unreliable. This is especially true for inpatient use, outpatient use, and emergency room use.

The second section of Table 7.2 presents the differences in mental health and substance abuse treatment expenditures by rural-urban status. As suggested in the utilization results, there is no significant difference in the total mental health and substance abuse treatment expenditures by rural-urban status. What is surprising in these results is that rural women pay less out of pocket for mental health and substance abuse treatment than their urban counterparts. While the magnitude of this difference diminished in 1997, rural women continued to incur lower out of pocket expenditures. This may be partially explained by the fact that rural women are slightly more likely to have public health insurance, which, on average, has more generous mental health and substance abuse treatment coverage than private health insurance. While the rural women pay less out of pocket for mental health and substance abuse treatment, rural women also have significantly lower incomes. Thus, the burden of out of pocket mental health and substance abuse treatment expenditures, or the percentage of income that is spent on mental health and substance abuse treatment, is similar for rural and urban women. While this difference may not be significant due to the extreme distribution of income and out of pocket expenditures,[4] it is relevant to policy as one examines the stressors and demands placed on rural women's health and the financial burdens that mental health and substance abuse treatment may cause rural women. As mentioned earlier, one must be cautious in the interpretation of these results for the same reasons as stated above and because the abnormal distribution of both expenditures and incomes is not taken into account in this simple measure.

To examine any differences in utilization and expenditures for rural minority women, controlling for potential confounding variables, multiple logistic regressions including a race-rural interaction were run as described in the methods section. Table 7.3 presents the odds ratios and p-values for the model where the outcome is a dichotomous measure equaling "1" if the woman had any mental health and/or substance abuse treatment utilization and "0" otherwise.

Married women were less likely than unmarried women to have had any mental health and/or substance abuse treatment during the year. Hispanic non-Black women and African American women were significantly less likely than urban White women to have had any mental health and/or substance abuse treatment. While rural status and the rural-African American interactions are not significant alone, their interpretation is more complex and will be discussed below. The rural variable was inconsistent (positive effect in 1996 and negative effect in 1997) and nonsignificant in both years. This may be due to the definition of rural (non-MSA). Being uninsured all year significantly decreased the odds of a woman having any mental health and/or substance abuse treatment compared with those women with private health insurance (43 percent as compared with 55 percent, respectively). On the other hand, having only public health insurance increased the odds of utilization and this difference is significant in the larger 1997 sample.

TABLE 7.3   Logistic Regression of Any MHSA Utilization

	1996		1997	
	Odds Ratio	p value	Odds Ratio	p value
Married***	0.667	< .001	0.614	< .001
Hispanic non-Black**	0.640	.010	0.664	.008
African American***	0.401	< .001	0.381	< .001
White, other	Reference category			
Rural	1.130	.285	0.961	.728
Rural and African American	0.963	.910	0.872	.660
Rural and Hispanic	1.368	.368	1.518	.172
Uninsured	0.452	< .001	0.629	.003
Public only	1.007	.969	1.273	.046
Any private	Reference category			
Northeast	0.924	.539	0.819	.105
Midwest	1.018	.884	0.960	.715
South	1.068	.544	0.997	.974
West	Reference category			
< 100% poverty level	0.865	.376	0.959	.753
100 to 124% poverty level	0.869	.537	0.829	.275
125 to 199% poverty level	1.081	.613	0.950	.686
200 to 399% poverty level	1.054	.624	0.888	.210
400% or greater	Reference category			
Age***	1.115	< .001	1.129	< .001
Age-squared*	0.999	< .001	0.999	< .001
High school or greater*	1.304	.061	1.562	< .001
Fair or poor mental health***	8.702	< .001	8.318	< .001
Employed	0.773	.044	0.884	.215

*p < .05
**p < .01
***p < .001

Finally, the model showed no difference in likelihood of utilization by poverty status or region. There was a nonlinear age effect in that, as one ages, the likelihood of mental health and/or substance abuse treatment declines. In addition, those women who have a high-school degree or higher have significantly higher odds of obtaining mental health and/or substance abuse treatment compared with those women without a high-school degree. This result is expected since those with higher educational attainment are likely to invest more in their health or may have greater access to, and ability to use, the health care system. Perceived mental health status is a very strong predictor of mental health and substance abuse treatment. This could be interpreted to mean that those who feel the need for mental health treatment are more likely to receive it. On the other hand, since the data used in this study are cross-sectional, the analyses cannot test the direction of this relationship, since those who receive treatment may perceive their mental health status to be fair or poor.

Logistic regression models were developed using the same independent variables as reported in Table 7.3 to evaluate outcomes, i.e., 1) any prescription drug treatment or 2) any office-based treatment. The models were applied only to those women who reported any mental health and/or substance abuse treatment during the year. The results from these models were similar to those reported in Table 7.3. One difference found was that women in all regions were significantly more likely to use prescription drugs than women in the Western region.

In order to interpret the interaction coefficients, one must examine the effects of the sum of the interaction coefficient (rural multiplied by African American) as well as the individual dummy variables from which the interaction variable was constructed (rural, African American). This combination was developed and the odds ratios for rural African American women are presented in Table 7.4.

Controlling for age, poverty status, mental health status, and education level, being a rural African American woman is significantly associated with lower odds of receiving any mental health and/or substance abuse treatment (56 percent vs. 68 percent). The odds that the mental health treatment received is a prescription drug or an office-based visit is higher for rural African American women when compared with urban White women, but this difference is not significant in either year.

TABLE 7.4 Odds Ratios for Rural African American for MHSA Treatments

	1996		1997	
MHSA Outcome Modeled	Odds Ratio	p value	Odds Ratio	p value
Any Mental Health Utilization*	0.436	.007	0.319	.000
Any Prescription Drug	1.929	.557	0.569	.363
Any Office-Based	1.163	.839	1.493	.587

From models that control for age, region, poverty status, mental health status, employment, education and insurance, similar to Table 7.3.
*$p < .01$

Models examining total mental health and substance abuse treatment expenditures were also examined. No significant difference was seen in total mental health and/or substance abuse treatment expenditures for rural African American women. Rural African American women did incur significantly less out of pocket expense for mental health services than urban White women in 1996 ($225/ average per capita), but this difference did not exist in the 1997 data.

DISCUSSION

This analysis provides a description of the type of mental health and substance abuse services rural women utilize as well as the total amount of expenditures and amount paid out of pocket for these services. In general, rural women are more likely to be White, married, less educated, and living at lower poverty levels. In addition, rural women rely more on public health insurance or remain uninsured all year when compared with their urban counterparts. In this analysis, there was little difference in mental health status, mental health service utilization, or types of services used between rural and urban women. While rural women used a higher percentage of acute care services for mental health than urban women, these differences were not significant. Rural women, however, spent less out of pocket than their urban counterparts. but they spent an equal percentage of their income. We do not know if this is due to the service or treatment being purchased (are they using fewer specialty services?) or whether the difference is due to the generosity of the publicly provided mental health insurance in covering benefits. Finally, we see that rural African American women are less likely to have any mental health and/or substance abuse treatment than their urban White counterparts. It is important for future researchers and policy analysts to study why this occurs. Is this difference due to lack of supply of providers? Do rural African American women seek other, nonmedical establishments (such as clergy, friends, social support) for mental health and/or substance abuse treatment? Is there a difference in the prevalence of the disorders in rural and urban women, and do different ethnic groups perceive mental illness and substance abuse differently? Is the difference due to differences in the stigma attached to mental illness and substance abuse by different ethnic groups? This study cannot answer these questions, but future research should examine these issues, especially in rural minority populations.

The explanation of the difference in out of pocket expenditures is unclear. While this may reflect a lower quantity of services purchased, or a lower price in rural areas due to lower reimbursement rates, the lower out of pocket mental health and substance abuse treatment expenditures may be due to more generous insurance coverage or lower cost of services (more primary care visits versus specialists and inpatient treatment). Another explanation is that rural residents have a lower cost of living in general. Further research will be needed to answer these questions.

LIMITATIONS

There are several limitations in this analysis. First, while the data are nationally representative, when multiple predictors are added to the analysis, the resulting decrease in statistical power adversely affects our ability to discern group differences, especially for minorities. A possible solution to this problem is to pool several years of the MEPS data to increase the number of observations, thus increasing their predictive power. In addition, these data only allow rural status to be identified by MSA and region. MSA is not a precise enough measure for rural status and thus the analysis may not find any rural-urban differences due to the blurring of this measure.

Policy makers and researchers often overlook rural minority populations when collecting data or developing research. This makes it difficult to study this unique population unless one uses state or area data. When researchers focus on regional or state populations the generalizability of the results is limited. Therefore, national data on rural minority health needs to be collected.

Another limitation of this analysis is that mental health and substance abuse treatment services were identified based on ICD-9 and V codes from the event files in the MEPS data. MEPS data only allows for three primary diagnoses, which may not capture all mental health and/or substance abuse utilization. In addition, not all diagnoses reported in the event files are confirmed by the provider audits, and thus they rely on self-reported diagnosis. This may further bias the results in that many people will not report mental health and/or substance abuse related treatments due to the stigma attached to these diseases. Some may be concerned that severely dysfunctional people may not provide reliable self-reported diagnoses. Since these data represent the noninstitutionalized population, this issue may not be as much of a concern. MEPS also attempts to control for self-report diagnosis bias by random provider audits.

Finally, as mentioned throughout, this report is an exploratory analysis and while certain associations are explored, causal relationships cannot be determined with these cross-sectional data. The models developed were applied without controlling for selection bias that occurs in the choice of health insurance. This could bias the results. For example, women may be eligible for public health insurance (Medicaid and/or Medicare Disability Insurance) by virtue of being severely mentally ill or mentally disabled. Because this analysis does not model this choice, the estimated coefficients for the insurance variables and any variables correlated with these insurance variables may be biased. Also, the models do not control for the severity of mental illness, comorbidities, or any supply variables, which may affect the likelihood of utilization.

FUTURE WORK

Future work with the Medical Expenditure Panel data will include pooling several years of data in order to increase the power. In addition, future models will include measures for type of mental illness and substance abuse as well as other comorbidities in order to address the concerns regarding severity of illness addressed above. If possible, future models should examine the expenditures by payer class, such as Medicaid, Medicare, and private insurance to attempt to control for selection and fully model the unobserved heterogeneity.

CONCLUSION

Compared with urban White women, rural African American women are significantly less likely to have any mental heath and/or substance abuse utilization during the year, even when controlling for demographics and self-reported mental health status. Rural women spend less out of pocket for mental health and substance abuse treatment than their urban counterparts. This may be due to rural females relying more on publicly provided health insurance. When the economy weakens and there are less public funds available for health care, rural women are placed in a vulnerable state, not being able to obtain health insurance and thus not being able to afford health care. Future research needs to examine why rural African Americans, and African Americans in general, are less likely to use mental health and substance abuse treatment services. What are the barriers to obtaining treatment? Are the barriers due to lack of demand, lack of transportation, geographic inaccessibility, social or cultural factors, or supply problems? In addition, researchers need to examine which health care professionals, paraprofessionals, and support groups provide mental health and substance abuse treatment services in rural areas.

NOTES

1. Office-based settings are those encounters that primarily took place in clinics or offices supervised by physicians. These included physicians as well as nonphysicians. The nonphysicians included chiropractors, nurses, nurse practitioners, midwives, optometrists, podiatrists, physician assistants, physical therapists, occupational therapists, psychologists, social workers, or other medical providers.

2. Events included in event files for this analysis are office-based visits, inpatient, outpatient, and emergency room visits, and prescription drugs.
3. AHRQ has collapsed various ICD-9 and V codes into large clinical conditions categories. For this analysis, clinical condition codes identified as mental health and/or substance abuse were included.
4. Out of pocket MHSA expenditures and income have non-normal distributions and thus using a simple test of means is not the most appropriate measure.

REFERENCES

Kessler, R. C., McGonagle, K. A., Zhao, S., Nelson, C. B., Hughes, M., Eshleman, S., et al. (1994). Lifetime and 12-month prevalence of DSM-111-R psychiatric disorders in the United States. *Archives of General Psychiatry, 51*(1), 8–19.

Manning, W. G., & Mullahy, J. (2001). Estimating log models: To transform or not to transform? *The Journal of Health Economics, 20,* 461–94.

Murray, C. J. L., & Lopez, A. D. (Eds.). (1996). *The global burden of disease: A comprehensive assessment of mortality and disability from diseases, injuries, and risk factors in 1990 and projected to 2020.* Cambridge, MA: Harvard School of Public Health.

Ricketts, T. C., III (1999). *Rural health in the United States.* New York: Oxford University Press.

Ringel, J. S., & Sturm, R. (2001). Financial burden and out-of-pocket expenditures for mental health across different socioeconomic groups: Results from HealthCare for Communities. *The Journal of Mental Health Policy and Economics, 4*(3), 141–150.

Rhodes, A. E., Goering, P. N., To, T., & Williams, J. I. (2002). Gender and outpatient mental health service sse. *Social Science & Medicine, 54*(1), 1–10.

Rost, K., Zhang, M., Fortney, J., Smith, J., & Smith, R., Jr. (1998). Rural-urban differences in depression treatment and suicidality. *Medical Care, 36*(7), 1098–1107.

Rost, K., Smith, G. R., & Taylor, J. L. (1993). Rural-urban differences in stigma and the use of care for depressive disorders. *Journal of Rural Health, 9*(1), 57–62.

Salkever, D., Shinogle, J. A., & Goldman, H. (1999, December). Does managed care substitute for limits and cost-sharing in mental health coverage? Evidence from a national employer survey. *Psychiatric Services, 50*(12), 1631–1633.

Thomas, K. C., & Snowden, L. R. (2001). Minority response to health insurance coverage for mental health services. *The Journal of Mental Health Policy and Economics, 4*(1), 35–41.

U.S. Department of Health and Human Services (1999). *Mental health: A report of the surgeon general.* Rockville, MD: U.S. Public Health Service.

Yuen, E. J., Gerdes, J. L., & Gonzales, J. J. (1996, January). Patterns of rural mental health care: An exploratory study. *General Hospital Psychiatry, 18*(1), 14–21.

Chapter 8

Understanding Mental Health Service Use Among Rural Women

Sarah Gehlert, Kelly Kovac, In Han Song, and
S. Ann Hartlage

Despite advances in our ability to serve those with mental conditions, an alarming number of persons with mental illness go without treatment (U.S. Department of Health and Human Services, 1999). The ramifications of lack of treatment are great. The Burden of Disease Study conducted by the World Health Organization, the World Bank, and Harvard University found that mental illness ranks second among selected illness categories in the United States and other established world economies as a contributor to the overall burden of disease (Murray & Lopez, 1996). Only cardiovascular conditions exceeded mental illness in the study's calculations of burden of disease.

Rural women use mental health services at a significantly lower rate than do women living in other areas. Estimates are that approximately 15 million of the nation's 62 million rural residents have diagnosable mental or substance abuse disorders (Roberts, Battaglia, Smithpeter, & Epstein, 1999). This prevalence rate, according to recent national surveys of the prevalence of psychiatric disorders in the United States (Robins & Regier, 1991), does not differ appreciably from the rates of urban residents. Yet, urban dwellers are significantly more likely to use mental health care services than are their rural counterparts (Comer & Mueller, 1995; Holzer & Ciarlo, 2000).

Inquiry into the differential use of mental health services among rural and urban residents, though largely conceptual rather than empirical in nature, has implicated several characteristics of rural environments as potential barriers to the use of services. Hill and Fraser (1995) note that many rural residents consider mental health problems to be the domain primarily of the church and family and are, therefore, less likely than urban dwellers to seek assistance at mental health clinics and other public or private institutions. In short, they believe that problems should not be handled by strangers.

Another potential barrier to the use of mental health services is the stigma associated with having mental health problems. Rost, Smith, and Taylor (1993) found that rural residents with histories of mental disorders labeled those who sought professional help more negatively than did their urban counterparts. Likewise, Hoyt, Conger, Valde, and Weihs (1997) found persons living in rural areas to express significantly higher levels of stigma related to mental health care than did residents of urban areas. Stigma is likely heightened by an inability in rural areas to receive care without the awareness of other members of the community (Merwin, Goldsmith, & Manderscheid, 1995). Roberts and colleagues (1999) note, too, that isolation in rural areas not only produces threats to patient confidentiality through overlapping relationships, roles that may be in conflict, and altered therapeutic boundaries between providers, patients, and significant others, but also produces stress for providers who may have no professional colleagues with whom to consult.

Lack of ability to pay for services is a more tangible barrier to seeking mental health care. Higher rates of poverty and lower incomes among persons living in rural areas suggest financial barriers to treatment. Rural residents are more likely to live in poverty (Hartley, Quam, & Lurie, 1994) and are less likely to have insurance coverage for mental health care. The latter may be due in part to the increased likelihood of working in agriculture or for small-business employers who are less able to purchase insurance for their employees (Fox, Merwin, & Blank, 1995).

Government funding decisions may also impede the provision of affordable mental health care services for rural residents. Rohland and Rohrer (1998) found that Iowa counties with fewer residents, higher proportions of rural and elderly residents, and higher proportions of income from farms spent less money on mental health services. The public mental health system is often the only source of services for rural residents. Rural areas still bear the vestiges of the catchment area system that was established initially under the Community Mental Health Centers Act of 1963 and continued with the Mental Health Block Grant. Under this system, mental health service delivery is tied to state and local policy and revenue streams (Mohatt, 2000). This system presents problems because 1) funding for mental health services under state and local auspices has not kept up with inflation, and 2) attempts at cost containment have limited services almost exclusively to persons with serious mental illness. Prevention and early case identification services, services for persons with less severe disorders, and combined services for people with concomitant substance abuse and metal health disorders are the services least likely to be available in rural areas (Mohatt, 2000). Using multiple funding streams to provide services for persons with multiple needs in an environment where services are scarce creates major problems in rural areas.

Only 16 percent of Medicare recipients living in rural areas had access to a Medicare+Choice plan in their area in 2001, compared with 82 percent of urban residents (McBride & Mueller, 2003). Medicaid pays for acute mental health services provided by mental health or primary care providers. Fewer providers are available in rural areas and those who are available may be disinclined to accept Medicaid's lower reimbursement rates.

The provider of mental health care also varies along the rural to urban continuum. Rural areas have fewer specialized mental health care practitioners and services (Merwin, Goldsmith, & Mandersheid, 1995), especially in the least urbanized nonmetropolitan areas (Holzer, Goldsmith, & Ciarlo, 2000). In the absence of specialized services, a substantial portion of mental health care is provided by primary care practitioners or human service providers (Regier et al., 1993). This is a problem because these providers are less likely to be adequately trained to diagnose and treat mental health problems. Adding to the problem is the reality that even the training of mental health professionals is geared toward urban circumstances rather than the realities of rural life (Heyman & VandenBos, 1989).

The present study tested a theoretically derived explanatory model of mental health services use among rural women. The model was designed to assess whether women living in a rural county in the midwestern United States sought mental health care. The model, based on the Behavioral Model of Health Services Use (Anderson, 1968, 1995), used demographic and social data, attitudes toward seeking professional help for mental health problems, information on likely social support for mental health problems, level of insurance coverage, and perceived and evaluated mental health to understand mental health care use and determinants of use.

METHODS

Participants

A four-site probability sample of women of reproductive age in the midwestern United States and a subsample of women in the most rural of the four sites were the foci of the present study. The larger sample was made up of 1,474 women selected by probability sampling from four sites of the Women's Wellness Study, a large study comparing changes in women's health through time, i.e., Chicago and DeKalb County, Illinois, and St. Louis and Franklin County, Missouri.

Based on data from the 1990 U.S. census, both St. Louis, Missouri and Chicago, Illinois fit the Census Bureau's definition of an urbanized area (U.S. Census Bureau, 1995). Both DeKalb County, Illinois and Franklin County, Missouri likewise can be considered rural, because none of their populations live within urbanized areas. Franklin County can be considered the more rural of the two, based on estimates that 60% of its residents reside in rural areas versus 32% of the residents of DeKalb County (U.S. Census Bureau, 1995).

A clear pattern was noted in the Women's Wellness Study data in which the number of visits to physicians for mental health or substance abuse problems decreased as the percentage of rural residents increased (Franklin County, $M = 3.09$, $SD = 3.36$; DeKalb County, $M = 5.06$, $SD = 8.75$; St. Louis, $M = 14.70$, $SD = 17.07$; Chicago, $M = 18.88$, $SD = 18.82$; $F = 5.55$, $p = .002$). We gathered a subsample of 349 women from Franklin County, Missouri, to examine the determinants of rural mental health service use in greater depth. The subsample represented all women from Franklin County who had completed participation in the larger study as of May, 2001.

Procedure

As part of the larger study, women completed daily symptom and mood ratings in their homes for two consecutive menstrual cycles and underwent thorough psychiatric testing for past and current mental conditions. Psychiatric testing was completed during the follicular phase of the first of the two cycles.

In order to gather additional data to more completely operationalize the variables of the Behavioral Model of Health Services Use (Anderson, 1968, 1995), women from Franklin County, Missouri were sent a 36-item survey soliciting information not gathered in the initial study. Franklin County was selected for the additional survey because it was the most rural of the four Women's Wellness Study sites and was well known to the senior author.

Instruments and Variables

On the survey mailed to Franklin County residents, women were asked if they had ever been treated by a professional for difficulties in managing their lives, an emotional or nervous problem, or a drinking or drug problem. Responses were dichotomous ("yes" or "no").

The framework for predicting women's mental health service use was derived from the Behavioral Model of Health Services Use developed by Anderson (1968, 1995). The model has gone through three phases since its development by Anderson (1968, 1995). We followed the lead of Anderson and Aday (1978), who used the behavioral model to understand levels of health services use among a probability sample of 7,787 noninstitutionalized persons in the United States, because we, too, were attempting to predict health services use, specifically use of mental health services. Anderson and Aday (1978) were able to explain 22% of the variance in number of physician visits in a multiple regression model using 1) age, race, and education of head of household as *predisposing* variables; 2) family income, doctor visit insurance, number of doctors per 1,000 population, and if a particular doctor was seen as *enabling* variables; and 3) illness symptoms and perceived health as *need* variables.

Predisposing Factors

Anderson and Aday (1978) define predisposing factors as those that suggest service use based on demographic and social characteristics and beliefs about health services. In the present study, age, race, and education and attitudes toward seeking mental health services are considered predisposing. The Fischer-Turner Attitudes Toward Seeking Professional Psychological Help Scale (ATSPPHS) (Fischer & Turner, 1970), which consists of 29 items rated on a 4-point rating scale (0 = disagree, 1 = probably disagree, 2 = probably agree, and 3 = agree), was chosen to measure attitudes toward mental health service use, for two reasons. It is one of the few scales to measure views toward seeking mental health services, rather than attitudes toward mental illness. Second, the ATSPPHS has proved to be psychometrically sound. Reliability scores with high internal consistency were reported by its authors ($r = .86$) (Fischer & Turner, 1970). Test-retest reliability scores ranged from .86 at five days to .84 at two months. That it was possible to distinguish known groups of students who were seeing or had seen a professional about a difficulty from those who had not ($t = 3.30$ and $p < .001$ for males; $t = 4.73$ and $p < .0001$ for females) suggested high criterion validity.

Enabling Factors

Anderson and Aday (1978) considered personal resources and the availability of health services in the community to be enabling variables. Several variables were considered enabling in the present study. Insurance type and coverage was solicited in the mailed survey. Participants were asked whether they had insurance coverage and, if so, which type (private, Medicaid, or Medicare). A second item asked whether participant's insurance would likely cover (totally or partially) treatment for psychological or mental health problems. From these data and knowledge of the providers in Franklin County and the types of insurance coverage they accepted, we were able to derive the measure *level of insurance*. Potential scores ranged from 0 (no insurance coverage for mental health problems) to 4 (coverage for any mental health services available in Franklin County). Another variable considered to be enabling, participant's total family income, was solicited on the exit interview for the larger study.

Perceived social support, which we define as an individual's perception that others in the environment would provide tangible or intangible support should she develop mental or emotional problems, is considered a personal/family enabling variable. Two questions on the Women's Quality of Life Questionnaire (WOMQOL), a questionnaire designed for the larger study (Gehlert, Chang, Hartlage, & Bock, in press), were used to assess perceived social support for mental health problems. Participants from the Franklin County, Missouri subsample were also asked to indicate in three questions whether they perceived that they could rely on various people in their environments to help with mental health conflicts or problems. Scores ranged from 0, indicating low perceived support, to 5, reflecting high levels of perceived support.

Although *providers per 1,000 population* is a standard component of the Behavioral Model of Health Services Use (Anderson, 1965, 1995), we were not able to use it in our analyses. Statistics were available only at the county level, and therefore would have been the same for all women in the study. We did compute the distance for each woman in the study to the next closest provider of mental health services. Scores ranged from fractions of a mile to 20 miles.

Need Factors

The factors in this category in the 1970s version of Behavioral Model of Health Services Use include illness symptoms as well as perceived health (Anderson & Aday, 1978). In the present study, illness symptoms became lifetime number of Axis I or Axis II diagnoses, which we termed *evaluated mental health*. Women in the original study underwent psychiatric testing for past and current Axis I disorders with an instrument appropriate for their age. Women age 13 to 17 years were given the Schedule for Affective Disorder and Schizophrenia for School-Age Children Epidemiologic Version-5 (K-SADS-E) (Chambers et al., 1985). Women between the ages of 18 and 55 years underwent testing using the Structured Clinical Interview for DSM-IV Axis I Disorders-Non-Patient Edition (SCID-I/NP) (First, Spitzer,

Gibbon, & Williams, 1996). Axis II disorders were assessed using the International Personality Disorder Examination (IPDE) (Loranger, Hirschfield, Sartorius, & Regier, 1991). Research assistants who received extensive training conducted the assessments. Inter-rater reliability scores were high (Kappa = 0.94, p = .03).

We were able to specify perceived health as *perceived mental health* by examining scores on 12 items on the WOMQOL. Four items were from each of three domains: mood, anxiety, and overall mental health. Scores from 0 through 3 were considered poor, and those from 4 through 6, 7 through 9, and 10 through 12 were considered fair, moderate, and excellent, respectively.

Analyses

Data analysis was conducted on the univariate, bivariate, and multivariate levels. Univariate and bivariate analyses were conducted to explore the structure of data. Logistic regression analyses were conducted to test the study's central research question. Variables were entered into the model according to our *a priori* conceptualization of mental health services use adapted from the Behavioral Model of Health Services Use (Anderson, 1968, 1995; Anderson & Aday, 1978). As such, need variables were entered first, then enabling factors, and lastly predisposing factors (see Instruments and Variables above). Each independent variable was treated as the dependent variable in a model with all other independent variables as predictors to detect multicollinearity (Menard, 2002). The adequacy of the final model was assessed using the Hosmer and Lemeshow goodness-of-fit test (Hosmer & Lemeshow, 1989), in which predicted probabilities were compared with those observed.

RESULTS

Completed surveys were returned by 155 women from Franklin County, Missouri, yielding a response rate of 49%. Twenty-nine surveys were returned by the post office as undeliverable; one blank survey form was returned by a participant. The mean age of the 155 responders was 35.9 years (*SD* = 9.4). Ages ranged from 15 to 56 years.

The 155 responders from Franklin County, Missouri (see Table 8.1) represented 2000 Decennial Census data for Franklin County (Missouri Census Data Center, n.d.) on a range of key demographic variables, such as age, ethnicity, and socioeconomic status. The percentages of ethnicity (i.e., 97.3 White, 0.7% American Indian, 0.7% Middle Eastern, 0.7% Hispanic, and 0.7% Asian/Pacific Islander) closely mirror percentages for the county as a whole (97.5% White, 0.9% Black, 0.2% American Indian, 0.7% Hispanic, 0.3% Asian/Pacific Islander, and 0.3% some other race). The median age for the sample of 37 years is close to the median age of 35.8 years reported for the county. Likewise, the percentage of women in the study receiving Medicaid (7.9%) is very close to that of Franklin County residents between the ages of 15 and 54 (8.1%).

Nonresponders to the study did not differ appreciably from either responders or county residents. They were slightly 1) younger ($M = 33.5$, $SD = 08.9$); 2) more ethnically diverse (90.7% White, 1.7% Black, 0.6% American Indian, 1.2% Hispanic, 0.6% Middle Eastern, 2.3% Biracial, and 0.6% some other race); and 3) less affluent (1.7% < $3,000, 1.7% $3,000–9,999, 4.1% $10,000–19,999, 5.2% $20,000–29,999, 15.1% $30,000–39,999, 16.3% $40,000–49,999, 12.8% $50,000–59,999, 17.4% $50,000–59,999, 16.9% $60,000–69,999, 8.7% did not know or refused to answer). The mean number of visits to physicians for mental health or substance abuse problems of nonresponders was almost identical to that of responders ($M = 3.0$, $SD = 2.4$ for nonresponders versus $M = 3.1$, $SD = 3.4$ for responders).

When lifetime Axis I diagnoses on the SCID or K-SADS-E and Axis II on the IPDE were considered, 95 women (64.2%) in the rural sample met diagnostic criteria. Of these women, 54 (56.8%) reported having received treatment for mental health problems at some time in their lives.

Results of logistic regression analysis can be found in Table 8.2. Evaluated health ($OR = 1.91$, 95% $CI = 1.39–2.64$, $p < .001$), ATSPPHS ($OR = 1.09$, 95% $CI = 1.01–1.17$, $p = .03$), age ($OR = 1.05$, 95% $CI = 1.00–1.11$, $p \leq .05$), and perceived health ($OR = 0.81$, 95% $CI = 0.68–0.97$, $p = .02$) were all positively and significantly associated with mental health services use. Collinearity among independent variables was low, with none obtaining an R^2 greater than 0.26 when used as the dependent variable in models with the other independent variables as predictors. The Hosmer and Lemeshow (1989) goodness-of-fit test

TABLE 8.1   Demographics of Study Sample

Characteristics	N	%
Race		
White	142	97.3
Latino	1	0.7
American Indian	1	0.7
Asian/Pacific Islander	1	0.7
Middle Eastern	1	0.7
Total family income		
< $3000	0	0.0
$3000–9999	4	2.9
$10000–19999	8	5.8
$20000–29999	12	8.8
$30000–39999	24	17.5
$40000–49999	27	19.7
$50000–59999	28	20.4
> 60000	34	24.8
Employment		
employed	96	66.7
unemployed	6	4.2
student	15	10.4
homemaker	24	16.7
other	3	2.1
Education		
less than 9 years of school	3	2.0
some high school (9 to 11 years)	15	10.3
high school graduate	28	19.2
some college or technical school	55	37.7
college graduate	32	21.9
post graduate education, no higher degree	5	3.4
graduate degree	8	5.5
Marital status		
married	100	68.0
single, living alone	22	15.0
single, living with partner	10	6.8
separated or divorced	15	10.2

TABLE 8.2 Logistic Regression Analysis: Factors Associated with Mental Health Services Use

Factor	Odds Ratio (95 Percent CI)	P value
Evaluated mental health	1.91 (1.39–2.64)	< .0001
ATSPPHS[1]	1.09 (1.01–1.17)	.03
Age	1.05 (1.00–1.11)	.05
Perceived mental health	0.81 (0.68–0.97)	.02
Level of insurance	1.36 (0.82–2.28)	ns
Distance from provider	1.08 (0.99–1.17)	ns
Perceived social support	1.01 (0.62–1.63)	ns
Education	0.98 (0.67–1.43)	ns
Income	0.86 (0.64–1.15)	ns

Note: CI = confidence interval, ns = not statistically significant at the $p \leq .05$ level.
[1]ATSPPHS = Fischer-Turner Attitudes Toward Seeking Professional Psychological Help Scale.

produced a p value of .55, indicating that the model fit the data reasonably well.

More simply put, women with Axis I or II diagnoses (i.e., those with evaluated mental health conditions) had 1.91 higher odds of receiving mental health services than women without Axis I or II diagnoses. Women with more favorable attitudes toward seeking mental health services, as measured by their scores on the ATSPPHS, had 1.09 higher odds of receiving mental health services than women with less favorable attitudes. Older women had 1.05 higher odds than younger women of receiving mental health services. Women who perceived themselves as being mentally healthy (i.e., had higher perceived mental health) had 1.24 lower odds of receiving mental health services than women who did not perceive themselves as mentally healthy.

DISCUSSION

Mental health services use in our rural county was well modeled by using a modified version of the Behavioral Model of Health Services Use (Anderson, 1968, 1995). In fact, the fit of our model was slightly better in trying to explain levels of health services use among a large national probability sample of noninstitutionalized persons than that obtained by Anderson and Aday (1978) using multiple regression. This may be due to our focus on a more specific concept, mental health services use, and our ability to gain specific information about aspects of mental health services delivery in Franklin County. Anderson (1995) notes that relationships are likely to be stronger when focusing on a particular disease and needs and services specific to that disease than when trying to relate general health beliefs to global measures of need and measures of services received.

Need variables, namely evaluated and perceived mental health, and predisposing variables, namely ATSPPHS and age, were more strongly associated with mental health services use than were enabling variables. No enabling variable was found to be significantly associated with health services use in our model. Although in Anderson and Aday's (1978) model total family income likewise failed to achieve significance, insurance for doctor's visits was found to be weakly but significantly associated with physician visits. That our level of insurance variable was not significantly associated with seeking mental health services may indicate that need and attitudes are so salient in the decision of whether to seek services that individuals never get to the point of making the decision based on whether they can pay for services.

Evaluated mental health was most strongly associated with mental health services use. This is certainly not surprising. One would expect the presence of symptoms of mental conditions to be an impetus toward seeking services. It remains difficult then to understand why 43.2% of women with objectively evaluated mental or substance abuse conditions, who presumably experienced symptoms that were not invisible to those around them, went without formal services. Although Anderson and Aday's (1978) model had no objectively determined measure of health problems, the number of symptoms reported by respondents in the past year best predicted number of physician visits. This is congruent with our finding that women who perceived their mental health as better were less likely to receive services.

If women are at some level aware that they have problems and are not significantly impeded by whether they can pay for mental health services, what then prevents them from seeking services? In the present study, attitudes toward seeking mental health services were variables strongly associated with services use. Our rural women had less favorable attitudes toward seeking mental health services than the vast majority of other groups for whom published norms could be found, e.g., $M = 48.7$, $SD = 7.0$ versus $M = 63.2$, $SD = 11.8$ for college females in the ATSPPHS normative sample (Fischer & Turner, 1970). It is likely that these less favorable attitudes toward seeking mental health services at least in part account for the high percentage of women who did not seek services.

Although distance from provider was not associated significantly with mental health services use in logistic regression analysis, its mean differed among the groups of women with and without diagnoses and with and without treatment (Dx/No Tx, $M = 2.3$, $SD = 4.1$; No Dx/No Tx, $M = 4.3$, $SD = 5.4$; Dx/Tx, M = 4.4, $SD = 1.7$; No Tx/Dx, M = 7.3, $SD = 5.2$; F 2.7, $p < .05$). Interestingly, women who had evaluated Axis I or Axis II disorders and had not been in for treatment lived significantly closer to mental health providers. Seeking services close to home increases the odds that others will be aware that a person is seeking mental health services, as has been suggested by Merwin, Goldsmith, and Manderscheid (1995). This awareness may lead to stigmatization. Paradoxically, in rural environments, living in close proximity to a mental health provider may be more of a barrier to treatment than living at a greater distance. It may be the case that our measure, *distance from provider,* may in fact be capturing *perception of stigma.*

The present study, though limited in scope to one Midwestern county, provides evidence of the pervasiveness of negative attitudes toward the seeking of mental health services by rural women and suggests that public health initiatives aimed at changing attitudes might increase rates of treatment among rural women with mental and substance abuse problems. Repeating the study in other rural locales, especially those with greater ethnic diversity, would ensure the generalizability of these findings and would allow for the further exploration and identification of the attitudes that serve as the most significant barriers to seeking services. Further study of how the symptoms of women with Axis I or Axis II diagnoses affect their lives and the lives of their significant others is warranted as is research on the extent and types of treatment provided through less formal networks. This information, some of which might be best collected using qualitative methods, would likely allow more effective interventions to be designed.

REFERENCES

Anderson, R. M. (1968). *Behavioral model of families' use of health services.* Research Series No. 25. Chicago, IL: Center for Health Administration Studies, University of Chicago.

Anderson, R. M. (1995). Revisiting the behavioral model and access to medical care: Does it matter? *Journal of Health and Social Behavior, 36*(1), 1–10.

Anderson, R., & Aday, L. A. (1978). Access to medical care in the U.S.: Realized and potential. *Medical Care, 16*(7), 533–546.

Chambers, W. J., Puig-Antich, J., Hirsch, M., Paez, P., Ambrosini, P. J., Tabrizi, M. A., et al. (1985). The assessment of affective disorders in children and adolescents by semi-structured interview: Test-retest reliability of the Schedule for Affective Disorders and Schizophrenia for School-Age Children, present episode version. *Archives of General Psychiatry, 42*(7), 696–702.

Comer, J., & Mueller, K. (1995). Access to health care: Urban-rural comparisons from a Midwestern agricultural state. *Journal of Rural Health, 11*(2), 128–136.

First, M. B., Spitzer, R. L., Gibbon, M., & Williams, J. B. W. (1996). Structured Clinical Interview for DSM-IV Axis 1 Disorders-Non-Patient Edition (SCID I/NP, Version 2.0). New York: New York State Psychiatric Institute, Biometrics Research.

Fischer, E. H., & Turner, J. L. (1970). Orientations toward seeking professional help: Development and research utility of an attitude scale. *Journal of Consulting and Clinical Psychology, 35,* 79–90.

Fox, J., Merwin, E., & Blank, M. (1995). De facto mental health services in the rural south. *Journal of Health Care for the Poor and Underserved, 6,* 434–468.

Gehlert, S., Chang, C-H., Hartlage, S. A., & Bock, D. R. (in press). The development and validation of the Women's Quality of Life Questionnaire (WOMQOL). *The Journal of Clinical Epidemiology.*

Hartley, D., Quam, L., & Lurie, N. (1994). Urban and rural differences in health insurance and access to care. *Journal of Rural Health, 10*(2), 98–108.

Heyman, S. R., & VandenBos, G. R. (1989). Developing local resources to enrich the practice of rural community psychology. *Hospital and Community Psychiatry, 40,* 21–23.

Hill, C. E., & Fraser, G. J. (1995). Local knowledge and rural mental health reform. *Community Mental Health Journal, 31,* 553–586.

Holzer, C. E., III, & Ciarlo, J. A. (2000). Mental health services utilization in rural and non-rural areas. *Journal of the Washington Academy of Sciences, 86*(3), 49–57.

Holzer, C. E, III, Goldsmith, H. F., & Ciarlo, J. A. (2000). The availability of health and mental health providers by population density. *Journal of the Washington Academy of Sciences, 86*(3), 25–33.

Hosmer, D. W., & Lemeshow, S. (1989). *Applied logistic regression.* New York: John Wiley and Sons.

Hoyt, D. R., Conger, R. D., Valde, J. G., & Weihs, K. (1997). Psychological distress and help seeking in rural America. *American Journal of Community Psychology, 25,* 449–470.

Loranger, A. W., Hirschfeld, R. M. A., Sartorius, N., & Regier, D. A. (1991). The WHO/ADAMHA international pilot study of personality disorders: Background and purpose. *Journal of Personality Disorders, 5,* 296–306.

McBride, T. D., & Mueller, K. J. (2003). *Inequitable access: Medicare+Choice program fails to serve rural America.* Retrieved August 22, 2003, from http://www.rupri.org/publications/archive/pbriefs/PB2002-2/PB2002-2.PDF

Menard, S. (2002). *Applied logistic regression analysis.* Thousand Oaks, CA: Sage.

Merwin, E. I., Goldsmith, H. F., & Manderscheid, R. W. (1995). Human resource issues in rural mental health services. *Community Mental Health Journal, 31,* 525–537.

Missouri Census Data Center (n.d.). *Demographic Profile 1, 2000 Census.* Retrieved July 25, 2001, from http://mcdc2.missouri.edu/websas/dp1_2k menus/mo

Mohatt, D. F. (2000). Access to mental health services in frontier America. *Journal of the Washington Academy of Sciences, 86*(3), 35–47.

Murray, C. J. L., & Lopez, A. D. (Eds.). (1996). *The global burden of disease: A comprehensive assessment of mortality and disability from diseases, injuries, and risk factors in 1990 and projected to 2020.* Cambridge, MA: Harvard School of Public Health.

Regier, D. A., Narrow, W. E., Rae, D. S., Manderscheid, R. W., Locke, B. Z., & Goodwin, F. K. (1993). The de facto U.S. mental and addictive disorders system: Epidemiologic catchment area prospective 1-year prevalence rates of disorders and services. *Archives of General Psychiatry, 50*(2), 85–94.

Roberts, L. W., Battaglia, J., Smithpeter, M., & Epstein, R. S. (1999). An office on Main Street: Health care dilemmas in small communities. *Hastings Center Reports, 29*(4), 28–37.

Robins, L. N., & Regier, D. A. (1991). *Psychiatric disorders in America: The Epidemiologic Catchment Area study.* New York: The Free Press.

Rohland, B. M., & Rohrer, J. E. (1998). Capacity of rural community mental health centers to treat serious mental illness. *Community Mental Health Journal, 34*(3), 261–273.

Rost, K., Smith, G. R., & Taylor, J. L. (1993). Rural/urban differences in stigma and the use of care for depressive disorders. *Journal of Rural Health, 9*(1), 57–62.

U.S. Census Bureau. (1995). *Urban and rural definitions.* Retrieved November 6, 2001, from http://www.census.gov/population/censusdata/urdef.txt

U.S. Department of Health and Human Services. (1999). *Mental Health: A Report of the Surgeon General.* Rockville, MD: U.S. Department of Health and Human Services, Substance Abuse and Mental Health Services Administration.

Chapter 9

Behavioral Risk Factors, Chronic Diseases, Health Care Access, and Health Status of Rural American Indian Women in Oklahoma

Janis E. Campbell, Zoran Bursac, and Lisa Perkins

INTRODUCTION

American Indians have decreased life expectancy and disproportionately high rates of morbidity associated with numerous health prob-

This research was supported by a grant from the Centers for Disease Control and Prevention to the Oklahoma State Department of Health (Grant Number U50-CCU617413-03). The authors would like to acknowledge and thank the American Indian people who participated in this survey. The authors acknowledge the assistance and cooperation of the Absentee-Shawnee, Chickasaw, Choctaw, Cherokee, Cheyenne-Arapaho, Pawnee, Seminole, Wichita, and Affiliated American Indian communities. The authors also wish to thank the Indian Health Care Resource Center of Tulsa for their contribution to the project. Many thanks to the REACH 2010 program staff and steering committee. They made this process run smoothly through their input and administrative support. Finally, thanks to OSDH BRFSS staff who made the data collection possible. The opinions expressed in this paper are those of the authors and do not necessarily reflect the views of the tribes or nations that participated.

lems (Indian Health Services, 2002; Rhoades, Hammond, Welty, Handler, & Amler, 1987). Chronic diseases are now the leading cause of death among Americans Indians, including cardiovascular disease (Gilliland, Owen, Gilliland, & Carter, 1997; Howard et al., 1995; Lee et al., 1990; Kattapong, Becker, & Gilliland, 1995; Welty et al., 1995), diabetes (Lee et al., 1995; Lee et al., 1994; Lee et al., 2002), respiratory disease (Rhoades, 1990; Samet, Key, Kutvirt, & Wiggins, 1980), and cancer (Centers for Disease Control and Prevention, 2003). Although cardiovascular disease mortality has historically been low among the American Indian populations, mortality is now increasing as lifestyles change (Kattapong, Becker, & Gilliland, 1995). While cardiovascular disease has become the leading cause of death, diabetes mortality has increased substantially over the past twenty years (Gilliland, Owen, Gilliland, & Carter, 1997; Lee et al., 1990). If this trend continues, diabetes may soon become the primary cause of death among American Indians (Gilliland, Owen, Gilliland, & Carter, 1997; Lee et al., 1990). Even though mortality rates among American Indians in the United States show a decreased risk of cancer (Centers for Disease Control and Prevention, 2003), Oklahoma mortality rates for cancer double when misclassification of race is taken into account. Moreover, cancer is the second leading cause of death among American Indians in the United States (Indian Health Services, 2002).

American Indians and Alaska Natives show increased risk in many major health status indicators (general health status, obesity, diabetes) and health risk behaviors (cigarette smoking, leisure-time physical activity) compared with other racial/ethic groups (Denny, Holtzman, & Cobb, 2003). American Indian/Alaska Native women in the United States show significantly worse health status and risk indicators—including poor health status, obesity, diabetes and cigarette smoking—compared with non-American Indian/Alaska Native women (Denny, Holzman, & Cobb, 2003).

Increasing mortality, risk factors, and poor health behaviors indicate the need for prevention efforts that focus on modifiable risk factors among American Indians, including hypertension, hypercholesterolemia, diabetes, obesity reduction, physical activity, and smoking (Welty et al., 1995). To assess the epidemiology of important behavioral risk factors, chronic diseases, health care access, and health status among rural American Indian women, data from a Behavioral Risk Factor Surveillance System (BRFSS) based survey for the Oklahoma REACH 2010 project were reviewed. These risk factors and chronic diseases are among the most important causes of morbidity and mortality in the United States today.

Racial and Ethnic Approaches to Community Health (REACH 2010) is part of the Department of Health and Human Services (DHHS) response to President Clinton's initiative to eliminate disparities in health status experienced by racial and ethnic minority populations in the following six priority areas by 2010: infant mortality, breast and cervical cancer, cardiovascular disease, diabetes, HIV infections and AIDS, and child and adult immunizations. For Phase I of the project, 35 nationwide sites were funded to carry out activities related to planning, data collection, and forming partnerships and coalitions. Competitive Phase II funding was awarded to 24 projects for implementation of planned interventions for each of the priority areas above.

The Oklahoma Native American REACH 2010 coalition was formed in May of 1999. Oklahoma was funded for Phase I in 1999 and for Phase II in 2000. The Oklahoma REACH 2010 project was designed to reduce disparities in cardiovascular disease and diabetes, and their risk factors among American Indians in Oklahoma through increased availability and promotion of physical activity on a community level. The REACH 2010 partnership includes members from Absentee-Shawnee Tribe of Oklahoma, Chickasaw Nation, Choctaw Nation, Cherokee Nation, Cheyenne-Arapaho Tribes of Oklahoma, Pawnee Nation of Oklahoma, Seminole Nation of Oklahoma, Wichita and Affiliated Tribes, Indians Health Care Resource Center of Tulsa, and the Oklahoma Sate Department of Health. While the statewide REACH 2010 project is coordinated through the Oklahoma Sate Department of Health, each of the nine community interventions are implemented and managed within the tribal or community settings.

Ethnic groups are often examined as a single, nonvarying entity. This is problematic because information about important subgroup differences, such as varying cultural and geographic norms by specific tribes, is not revealed. Excluding consideration of cultural differences among tribes often reduces the effectiveness of planning and delivery of health care services for these groups. The goal of this report is to discuss the health status of rural American Indian women in Oklahoma with respect to several chronic conditions, their major risk factors, health care access and use, and barriers to delivery of prevention services. Accurate analysis and understanding of health status and behavioral risk factors can help implement successful health promotion programs and public health interventions within American Indian tribes and communities. This study offers a unique opportunity to advance our understanding of the health of American Indian women by providing important information about the rural segment of the American Indian population in Oklahoma.

DATA COLLECTION AND METHODS

This analysis used data from two major sources: the Oklahoma REACH 2010 Behavioral Risk Factor Survey (REACH 2010 BRFS) and the Oklahoma Behavioral Risk Factor Surveillance System (BRFSS).

The BRFSS is an ongoing, state-based, random-digit dialed telephone survey of the noninstitutionalized adult population age 18 years and older that live in households. The survey is supported by the Centers for Disease Control and Prevention (CDC). The purpose of the BRFSS is to collect consistent, state-based data on preventive health practices and behavioral risks that are linked to chronic diseases, injuries, and preventable infectious diseases (Centers for Disease Control and Prevention, 1998). Through a series of monthly telephone interviews conducted according to the data collection protocol, states uniformly collect data on the risks and diseases that are the leading causes of morbidity and mortality in the United Sates. When aggregated and weighted, these data show the prevalence of risk behaviors and preventive health practices on an annual basis for both the United States and for each state or territory (Centers for Disease Control and Prevention, 1998). For the purposes of this report Oklahoma BRFSS data collected between January 1999 and December 2001 were used. Standard BRFSS protocols and analysis techniques were used. A total of 11,204 surveys were collected; 6,706 of respondents were women; 6,262 of these were non-American Indian/Alaska Native.

As a part of Phase I of the Oklahoma REACH 2010 project, a random-digit dialed telephone survey using a BRFSS-like instrument was completed as a community level planning and evaluation tool. These surveys were completed separately from the CDC-sponsored

Oklahoma BRFSS, but by the same interview staff using the same protocols. Data were collected from adults age 18 and older to address the issue of diabetes, cardiovascular disease, overweight and obesity, physical (in)activity, tobacco use, and other behavioral risk factors, as well as some intermediate outcomes relevant to the project objectives. The survey was designed to provide adequate regional and statewide estimates for these and other issues associated with American Indian population of Oklahoma and the REACH 2010 project.

The Oklahoma REACH 2010 BRFS collected 3,732 surveys from seven strata, using a disproportionate stratified sampling scheme with screening. Zip codes were used as the sampling unit for each stratum (Fig. 9.1). The seven strata were determined based on historical tribal location and REACH 2010 project community locations. Using zip codes in these seven strata, only 3.7 percent of the total American Indian population of Oklahoma was excluded from potentially being surveyed. This strategy dramatically decreased the number of phone numbers and phone calls needed. Screening questions were used to determine self-identified race and eligibility for the survey. The survey was conducted from January 2000 through January of 2001, with an estimated response rate of 82 percent.

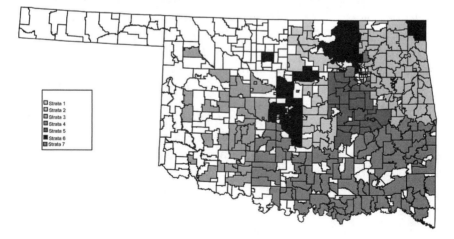

FIGURE 9.1   Zip code areas used for sampling in Oklahoma REACH 2010 Native American BRFS.

The Oklahoma REACH 2010 BRFS used selected questions from the year 2000 BRFSS questionnaire with the state specific screening questions and additional exercise questions from the Department of Epidemiology and Biostatistics and Department of Exercise Science at the School of Public Health, University of South Carolina in Columbia, South Carolina. Survey design and questions were approved by the Oklahoma REACH 2010 Steering Committee in October 1999.

The data were weighted to create statewide estimates for American Indians in Oklahoma. In order to create accurate statewide estimates, the data were weighted by the proportion of the American Indian 1990 population living in Oklahoma (U.S. Census Bureau, 1990). The data were weighted by sex and age categories using the age groups: 18–24, 25–64 by intervals of 10 years, over 64, as well as the different sampling from the seven strata. Neither the number of telephones in the household nor the number of adults was used since both are unreliable. The former does not adequately provide the distinct number of telephone numbers and may primarily reflect the number of instruments. The latter includes all races and is unreliable without more detailed information of whether adults are American Indians or not, particularly in Oklahoma where many American Indians reside in mixed-race households.

For this analysis 2,318 female respondents were divided into urban (N = 865) and rural (N = 1,453) groups. Urban respondents were those residing within any of the five Oklahoma Metropolitan Statistical Areas (MSAs), Enid, Lawton, Oklahoma City, Tulsa, and Fort Smith. Rural respondents included all others. For this report, only rural American Indian women were analyzed.

In this analysis rural American Indian women in Oklahoma were compared with Non-American Indian or Alaska Native women in Oklahoma. These data are from the Oklahoma REACH 2010 BRFS and Oklahoma BRFSS surveys unless otherwise stated. For most variables, prevalence rates and standard errors were provided. Observed differences were determined to be significant when p-values were less than .05.

RESULTS

Over half of American Indian women in Oklahoma (50.9 percent) live in rural areas; among Non-American Indian/Alaska Native Oklahoma women, 40.8 percent live in rural areas. The mean age for rural American Indian women was 44.2 compared with a mean age of 47.3 for Non-American Indian/Alaska Native Oklahoma women. This represents a statistically significant difference of three years. Among rural American Indian women in Oklahoma, 35.7 percent report their race as American Indian only; 61.4 percent report their race as American Indian and White, and 2.4 percent as American Indian and African American.

Oklahoma has 39 federally recognized tribes in the state and the second largest number of American Indians of any state (U.S. Census Bureau, 2000). In this survey 74 tribes were represented, including tribal members residing in Oklahoma whose tribal government headquarters are located outside of Oklahoma (e.g., Navaho). Among rural American Indian women in the survey, 47.2 percent of respondents were Cherokee, 18.0 percent Choctaw, 7.6 percent Creek, 5.9 percent Chickasaw, 3.3 percent Comanche, 2.7 percent Kiowa, and 1.6 percent Seminole. These proportions compared with 40.1 percent Cherokee, 16.6 percent Choctaw, 8.8 percent Creek, 5.2 percent Chickasaw, 1.7 percent Comanche, 2.0 percent Kiowa, and 2.6 percent Seminole in the overall population of Oklahoma in 2000 (U.S. Census Bureau, 2000). Among rural American Indian women, 21.5 percent understand an American Indian language, 11.3 percent were capable of speaking an American Indian language, and 5.5 percent speak an American Indian language regularly, such as at home or with relatives or friends.

American Indian women show no significant difference in educational attainment when compared with Non-American Indian/Alaska Native Oklahoma women overall (Table 9.1). In employment, when compared with Non-American Indian/Alaska Native Oklahoma women (Table 9.1), rural American Indian women showed an increased likelihood of unemployment (9.9 percent vs. 6.6 percent), but a decreased likelihood of retirement among employed rural American Indian women (16.3 percent vs. 20.6 percent). Rural American Indian women show significant and dramatic differences in household income compared with Non-American Indian/Alaska Native Oklahoma women (Table 9.1). They were significantly more likely to have a household income of less than $15,000 each year (23.0 percent vs. 14.5 percent), more likely to have income ranging from $15,000 to $34,999 (52.1 percent vs. 45.2 percent) and less likely to have income of $35,000 or more (24.9 percent vs. 40.3 percent)

TABLE 9.1 Demographic Characteristics of Rural American Indian and Non-American Indian/Alaska Native Women: Oklahoma 1999–2001

Characteristic	Rural AI Women[1]	S.E.	Non-AI/AN Oklahoma Women[2]	S.E.
Education				
Less than high school	16.3	1.10	14.8	0.54
High school	37.8	1.53	35.6	0.71
Some college	28.1	1.43	27.9	0.67
College graduate	17.8	1.21	21.3	0.61
Employment				
Employed	53.9	1.56	53.6	0.75
Homemaker	15.6	1.17	15.4	0.59
Retired	16.3*	1.07	20.6	0.58
Student	4.3	0.78	3.7	0.34
Unemployed	9.9*	0.91	6.6	0.38
Yearly household income				
Less than $15000 per year	23.0*	1.44	14.5	0.61
$15,000–34,999	52.1*	1.73	45.2	0.87
$35,000 or more	24.9*	1.49	40.3	0.86

1. Oklahoma REACH 2010 BRFSS
2. Oklahoma BRFSS 1999–2001
* significant at alpha .05

than Non-American Indian/Alaska Native Oklahoma women overall (Table 9.1).

Rural American Indian women were significantly more likely than Non-American Indian/Alaska Native Oklahoma women to currently smoke cigarettes (30.1 percent vs. 24.0 percent; Table 9.2). Rural American Indian women were significantly more likely to be overweight (53.6 percent compared with 46.4 percent) and obese (27.5 percent compared with 19.8 percent) than Non-American Indian/Alaska Native Oklahoma women (Table 9.2). On the positive side, rural American Indian women were significantly more likely to participate in physical activity or exercise than Non-American Indian/Alaska Native Oklahoma women overall (67.3 percent compared with 61.0 percent; Table 9.2). There were no significant differences in self-reported high cholesterol or high blood pressure (Table 9.2).

TABLE 9.2 Behavioral Risk Factors, Chronic Diseases, Health Care Access, and Health Status of Rural American Indian and Non-American Indian/Alaska Native Women: Oklahoma 1999–2001

Characteristic	Rural AI Women[1]	S.E.	Non-AI/AN Oklahoma Women[2]	S.E.
Risk factors				
Cigarette smoking[2]	30.1*	1.44	24.0	0.65
Overweight[2,3]	53.6*	1.58	46.4	0.80
Obese[2]	27.5*	1.39	19.8	0.62
Any exercise[2]	67.3*	1.46	61.0	0.74
High cholesterol[2]	29.0	1.66	27.9	0.75
High blood pressure[4]	27.0	1.35	25.6	0.79
Chronic diseases				
Gestational diabetes[2]	1.3	0.36	0.8	0.11
Diabetes[2]	10.6*	0.92	5.8	0.34
Heart disease or myocardial infarction[2]	2.4	0.42	1.6	0.16
Stroke[2]	3.3	0.52	2.5	0.21
Ever diagnosed with asthma[5]	19.0*	1.28	10.7	0.54
Current asthma[2]	13.3*	1.10	7.8	0.45
Health care access				
Health coverage of any kind[2]	89.8*	0.92	83.4	0.62
Checkup last 2 years[5]	10.6	1.07	11.3	0.60
Cholesterol not tested[2]	28.4*	1.49	22.9	0.68
Blood pressure 1 year or longer[6]	6.1*	0.79	3.3	0.54
Cost too much last year[5]	20.3*	1.26	11.4	0.62
Health status				
Limited[7]	24.5*	1.28	18.1	0.64
Mean days poor health limited activities[7]	11.3*	0.72	4.5	0.19
General health[2]				
Fair/poor	25.2*	1.31	17.8	0.55
Good	27.9	1.40	27.9	0.69
Excellent/very good	46.9*	1.58	54.3	0.76

1. Oklahoma REACH 2010 BRFSS
2. Oklahoma BRFSS 1999–2001
3. Includes obese
4. Oklahoma BRFSS 1999 and 2001
5. Oklahoma BRFSS 1999–2000
6. Oklahoma BRFSS 1999
7. Oklahoma BRFSS 2000–2001
* significant at alpha .05

When looking at self-reported chronic diseases two important diseases emerge. Rural American Indian women were significantly more likely than Non-American Indian/Alaska Native Oklahoma women to report having been diagnosed with diabetes (10.6 percent vs. 5.8 percent; Table 9.2). Rural American Indian women were also significantly more likely to have at one time been told they have asthma by a physician (19.0 percent vs. 10.7 percent) and to still have asthma (13.3 percent vs. 7.8 percent; Table 9.2). While the prevalence rates were higher, there was no significant difference between rural American Indian women and Non-American Indian/Alaska Native Oklahoma women in heart disease or myocardial infarction, stroke, or gestational diabetes (Table 9.2).

Preventive health behaviors include health care coverage as well as access to and use of preventive health services. Rural American Indian women (89.8 percent) were significantly more likely to have some kind of health coverage than Non-American Indian/Alaska Native Oklahoma (83.3 percent; Table 9.2). This health care coverage includes health insurance, prepaid plans such as HMOs, government plans such as Medicare or Medicaid, as well as Indian Health Services, Tribal Health Services, or an urban health clinic. While this issue will be addressed in the discussion, it should be stressed that while American Indian women have access to Indian Health Services and Tribal Health Services, this care is limited, in most cases due to funding disparities, and is not comprehensive. This is central to interpretation of findings since those unfamiliar with the Indian Health Service are often unaware of these issues and mistakenly equate this coverage to private full coverage health insurance. While not significantly different, 10.6 percent of rural American Indian women have not had a routine checkup in the last two years compared with 11.3 percent of Non-American Indian/Alaska Native Oklahoma women (Table 9.2). However, significantly more rural American Indian women had not had their blood pressure taken (6.1 percent) in the last year compared with Non-American Indian/Alaska Native Oklahoma women (3.3 percent; Table 9.2). Additionally, significantly more rural American Indian women (28.4 percent) had never had their cholesterol tested compared with Non-American Indian/Alaska Native Oklahoma women (22.9 percent; Table 9.2). Finally, almost one in five rural American Indian women (20.3 percent) needed medical care but could not get it because of cost as compared with 11.4 percent of Non-American Indian/Alaska Native Oklahoma women (Table 9.2).

Health status includes self-reported general health, limitations of activities, and the number of days of poor health limited activities. One in four rural American Indian women (24.5 percent) reported that they have limitations because of a health impairment or health problem compared with 18.1 percent of Non-American Indian/Alaska Native Oklahoma women (Table 9.2). Among these women with limitations, rural American Indian women had poor physical or mental health keeping them from doing their usual activities, such as self-care, work, or recreation for an average of 11.3 days per month compared with 4.5 days per month among Non-American Indian/Alaska Native Oklahoma women (Table 9.2). Finally, rural American Indian women were significantly less likely than Non-American Indian/Alaska Native Oklahoma women to report their health as very good or excellent (46.9 percent vs. 54.3 percent); conversely they were also significantly more likely to report their health as fair or poor (25.2 percent vs. 17.8 percent; Table 9.2).

DISCUSSION

Disparities exist for American Indian women from Non-American Indian/Alaska Native Oklahoma in several important aspects of chronic diseases, their major risk factors, and health care access and use. Rural American Indian women in Oklahoma were at increased risk of daily cigarette smoking and being overweight and obese compared with non-American Indian/Alaska Native Oklahoma women. Cigarette smoking acts with other risk factors to greatly increase the potential for chronic obstructive pulmonary disease (COPD), coronary heart disease, and several types of cancer including lung, mouth, larynx, bladder, cervix, uterus, and pancreas. Because of the increased prevalence of cigarette smoking among rural American Indian women the risk of onset of these diseases is higher among this population.

Body Mass Index (BMI) is a common measure expressing the relationship (or ratio) of weight to height. BMI is a mathematical formula in which a person's body weight in kilograms is divided by the square of his or her height in meters, i.e., $wt/(ht^2)$. The BMI is more highly correlated with body fat than any other indicator of height and weight. Individuals with a BMI of 25 to 29.9 are considered to be overweight, while individuals with a BMI of 30 or more are considered to be obese. Overweight and obese individuals are at increased risk for physical ailments such as high blood pressure, high blood cholesterol, Type 2 (non-insulin dependent) diabetes, insulin resistance, glucose intolerance, hyperinsulinemia, coronary heart disease, angina pectoris, congestive heart failure, stroke, gallstones, gout, osteoarthritis, obstructive sleep apnea and respiratory problems, some types of cancer (such as endometrial, breast, prostate, and colon), complications of pregnancy, poor female reproductive health (such as menstrual irregularities, infertility, irregular ovulation), bladder control problems (such as stress incontinence), uric acid nephrolithiasis, and psychological disorders (such as depression, eating disorders, distorted body image, and low self-esteem) (National Institutes of Health, 1998; Stunkard & Wadden, 1993). Again, because of increased prevalence of overweight and obesity, rural American Indian women are at increased risk for all of these conditions.

Because of these increased risk factors it comes as no surprise that rural American Indian women are disproportionately affected by high prevalence of diabetes and asthma. Diabetes is a major risk factor for cardiovascular disease among American Indians. The high current prevalence of diabetes as well as the major risk factors, suggests that mortality from diabetes and cardiovascular diseases may continue to increase unless vigorous efforts for primary and secondary prevention are urgently implemented. It is also important to note that the lack of significant differences in prevalence of heart disease or myocardial infarction and stroke does not necessarily represent a true lack of increased risk for these conditions. As with all potentially acute diseases all three conditions may only be found immediately prior to or after death. The decreased access to comprehensive care for this population as well as the limited access to acute hospital care in rural settings suggests that rural American Indian women may be at increased risk of dying from these conditions and thus showing lower rates of prevalence. In short, more analysis is needed on survival of myocardial infarction and stroke among American Indian women before a determination of the risk for these conditions can be made.

The outcomes presented in this analysis show large health burdens for American Indian women. Some of the risk factors, however, associated with them are potentially reversible. For example, the Diabetes Prevention Program Research Group recently demonstrated through a large clinical trial that moderate lifestyle changes including weight loss and weekly physical activity participation can potentially reduce diabetes incidence by 58 percent (Knowler et al., 2002). While rural American Indian women are already more likely to participate in exercise, there were still well over 30 percent who did not participate in any leisure time physical activity, and more who are not participating enough to benefit their health.

The apparent contradiction between the higher rates of health care coverage and the significantly lower rates of cholesterol testing and not having seen a physician in the last year because of the cost is important for several reasons. First, Indian Health Services and Tribal Health Services are available for the vast majority of rural American Indian women. According to our data, screening services are being underutilized. Second, it should be noted that while Indian Health Services and Tribal Health Services provide health care to American Indians it is not comprehensive. Services are contingent on available funding and the level of services offered often differs by geographic area. This is reflected in the over 20 percent of rural American Indian women who, because of cost issues, did not receive needed care.

The results of this report are subject to at least three limitations. First, these data are self-reported and, thus, cannot be verified. They are subject to recall bias. However, self-report measures have been the subject of numerous reliability and validity studies that suggest limited bias (Nelson, Powell-Griner, Town, & Kovar, 2003; Shea, Stein, Lantiqua, & Basch, 1991). These studies include BRFSS-specific questions that are the basis for both data sources. A recent study compared BRFSS estimates with estimates from the face-to-face National Household Interview Survey (NHIS). It demonstrated that while estimates may differ within subgroups, the BRFSS provides overall estimates that are comparable to those from NHIS (Nelson, Powell-Griner, Town, & Kovar, 2003). Second, REACH 2010 BRFS and BRFSS are telephone-based surveys. Persons of low socioeconomic status, who are less likely to have been screened, are also less likely to have a telephone and thus may not be included. It is estimated that only 5 percent of Oklahomans overall and 21 percent of American Indians do not have residential phone service. Because of this lack of telephone access, the prevalence of specific risk factors, chronic diseases, health care access, and health status variables may be underestimated. Though accounted for through statistical weighting methods, this insufficiency can never quite be eliminated. One method that was applied during Phase I of the REACH 2010 project in Oklahoma was recruitment of more than 500 American Indian individuals without telephones in their household to complete the same survey over the phone to learn more about the differences between the two groups. Based on the matched data analysis performed on the two surveys we found several differences. Individuals without telephones were more likely to have diabetes and higher smoking and obesity rates, were more likely to use Indian or Tribal Health Services, and to have less education. We estimated that proportional inclusion of persons without telephones in the random survey would increase our estimates by 1–2 percentage points, depending on the measure of interest. Third, problems might be caused by language barriers. American Indian languages are still spoken as the primary language in many households. This is especially true among elders. Our survey data shows that a tribal language is spoken daily with relatives and friends in 5 percent of the American Indian households in Oklahoma.

Because of these increased risk factors and chronic diseases, it is not surprising that rural American Indian women exhibited a higher frequency of fair or poor health status and a higher number of limited activity days due to poor physical or mental health. All of this is despite the fact that rural American Indian women were more likely to have health coverage and were, on average, three years younger. These results complement several studies that have shown disproportional and increased risk of some chronic diseases among American Indians in Oklahoma (Howard et al., 1995; Lee et al., 1995; Lee et al., 2002). Further, we showed how risk factors, primarily smoking, being overweight, and physical inactivity, are commonly distributed among rural American Indian women, and that decreasing these risk factors needs to be the primary purpose of prevention programs. Physical activity, smoking cessation, lifestyle risk reduction, and health care access programs need to be made increasingly available to all American Indian women. It is important to note that barriers such as the lack of a physical environment conducive to health promotion are characteristic of many rural Native communities. Many Native communities do not have more than one grocery store, thus limiting the choices of food Native Americans can purchase. Many Native communities do not have access to either indoor or outdoor fitness facilities such as walking trails. Any program within the American Indian community will be successful and acceptable only if the program is planned and implemented by the community in conjunction with the funding source. This requires designating strategies that recognize the disparities in infrastructure as well as the specific risk and chronic disease patterns. The inclusion of communities in planning prevention activities and risk modification programs in both the urban and rural settings is crucial to the attitudes of acceptance toward prevention programs.

REFERENCES

Centers for Disease Control and Prevention (1998). *Behavioral risk factor surveillance system user's guide*. Atlanta, GA: U.S. Department of Health and Human Services.

Centers for Disease Control and Prevention (2003). Cancer mortality among American Indians and Alaska Native—United States, 1994–1998. *Morbidity and Mortality Weekly Report, 52*(30), 704–707.

Denny, C. F., Holtzman, D., & Cobb, N. (2003). Surveillance for health behaviors of American Indians and Alaska Natives: Findings from the Behavioral Risk Factor Surveillance System, 1997–2000. *Morbidity and Mortality Weekly Report, 52*(SS07), 1–13.

Gilliland, F. D., Owen, C., Gilliland, S. S., & Carter, J. S. (1997). Temporal trends in diabetes mortality among America Indians and Hispanics in New Mexico: Birth cohort and period effects. *American Journal of Epidemiology, 145,* 422–431.

Howard, B. V., Lee, E. T., Cowan, L. D., Fabsitz, R. R., Howard, W. J., & Oopik, A. J. (1995). Coronary heart disease prevalence and its relation to risk factors in American Indians: The Strong Heart Study. *American Journal of Epidemiology, 142,* 254–268.

Indian Health Services (2002). *Trends in Indian Health 1998–1999*. Rockville, MD: U.S. Department of Health and Human Services.

Kattapong, V., Becker, T., & Gilliland, F. (1995). Ischemic Heart Disease Mortality In American Indians, Hispanics, and Non-Hispanics Whites 1958–1992. *American Indian Culture and Research Journal, 19*(2), 31–43.

Knowler, W. C., Barrett-Connor, E., Fowler, S. E., Hamman, R. F., Lachin, J. M., Walker, E. A., et al. (2002). Reduction in the incidence of Type 2 diabetes with lifestyle intervention or Metformin. *New England Journal of Medicine, 346*(6), 393–403.

Lee, E. T., Howard, B. V., Savage, P. J., Cowan, L. D., Fabsitz, R. R., Oopik, A. J., et al. (1995). Diabetes mellitus and impaired glucose tolerance in three American Indian populations: The Strong Heart Study. *Diabetes Care, 18*(5), 599–610.

Lee, E. T., Lee, V. S., Lu, M., Lee, L. S., Russell, D., & Yeh, J. (1994). Incidence of renal failure in NIDDM: The Oklahoma Indian Diabetes Study. *Diabetes, 43*(4), 572–579.

Lee, E. T., Welty, T. K., Cowan, L. D., Wang, W., Rhoades, D. A., Devereux, R., et al. (2002). Incidence of diabetes in American Indians of three geographical areas: The Strong Heart Study. *Diabetes Care, 25*(1), 49–54.

Lee, E. T., Welty, T. K., Fabsitz, R., Cowan, L. D., Le, N. A., Oopik, A. J., et al. (1990). The Strong Heart Study: A study of cardiovascular disease in American Indians: Design and methods. *American Journal of Epidemiology, 132*(6), 1141–1155.

National Institutes of Health (1998). Clinical Guidelines on the Identification, Evaluation, and Treatment of Overweight and Obesity in Adults (NIH Publication No. 98-4083). Washington, DC: Author.

Nelson, D. E., Powell-Griner, E., Town, M., & Kovar, M. G. (2003). A comparison of national estimates from the National Health Interview Survey and the Behavioral Risk Factor Surveillance System. *American Journal of Health, 93*(8), 1335–1341.

Rhoades, E. R. (1990). The major respiratory diseases of American Indian. *American Review of Respiratory Disease, 141*, 595–600.

Rhoades, E. R., Hammond, J., Welty, T. K., Handler, A. O., & Amler, R. W. (1987). The Indian burden of illness and future health interventions. *Public Health Reports, 102*, 361–368.

Samet, J. M., Key, C. R., Kutvirt, D., & Wiggins, C. L. (1980). Respiratory disease mortality in New Mexico's American Indians and Hispanics. *American Journal of Public Health, 70*(5), 492–497.

Shea, S., Stein, A. D., Lantiqua, R., & Basch, C. E. (1991). Reliability of the Behavioral Risk Factor Survey in a triethnic population. *American Journal of Epidemiology, 133*(5), 489–500.

Stunkard, A. J., & Wadden, T. A. (Eds.). (1993). *Obesity: Theory and therapy* (2nd ed.). New York: Raven Press.

U.S. Census Bureau (1990).

U.S. Census Bureau (2000).

Welty, T. K., Lee, E. T., Yeh, J., Cowan, L. D., Go, O., Fabsitz, R. R., et al. (1995). Cardiovascular disease risk factors among American Indians: The Strong Heart Study. *American Journal of Epidemiology, 142*(3), 269–287.

Chapter 10

The Role of Resources in the Emotional Health of African American Women: Rural and Urban Comparisons

Paula Y. Goodwin, Sharon Wallace Williams, and Peggye Dilworth Anderson

INTRODUCTION

To date the plight of rural African Americans is not well understood. Most studies regarding African Americans have focused on samples of urban African Americans because they are greater in numbers and more accessible to researchers than their rural counterparts. According to the 1997 Current Population Survey, about 15% of the total African American population lives in rural areas. Rural African Americans are geographically concentrated, with over 90% of them residing in Alabama, Arkansas, Georgia, Louisiana, Mississippi, North Carolina, South Carolina, Tennessee, Texas, or Virginia (Wimberly & Morris, 1996). Furthermore, about 20% of rural African Americans reside in "Black" counties, which are defined as counties with at least one third or more of its population consisting of African Americans (Cromartie, 1999).

Black counties and other minority counties are often plagued by severe, persistent poverty and underdevelopment which makes them comparable to urban areas in many ways and equally in need of research and intervention (Conger, 1997). O'Hare and Curry-White (1992) describe a growing rural underclass (defined as individuals who have not completed high school, receive public assistance, are never-married mothers, or are long-term unemployed males) that rivals the urban underclass populations. The majority (65%) of persons defined as rural underclass are African Americans who reside in the South (Smith, 1998). Therefore, many of the factors associated with depressive symptoms, such as financial strain and low educational attainment, are prevalent in both urban and rural African American communities. The purpose of this study is to examine and compare depressive symptoms among urban and rural African American women by exploring the roles of personal, social, and economic resources in emotional health.

AFRICAN AMERICANS AND MENTAL HEALTH

Epidemiological studies of noninstitutionalized community samples report the prevalence rates of depressive symptoms among African Americans to be between 20 and 30 percent (Brown, 1990). Depressive symptoms can include feelings of sadness, negative perceptions of self, helplessness, and disturbances in sleep, appetite, and sexual interest. Oftentimes, depressive symptoms make it difficult for persons to perform family and work duties and, in some instances, may lead to major depression. Several demographic factors have been associated with depressive symptomatology. Among them are lower educational levels and being impoverished (Brown, 1990; Dilworth-Anderson, 1998). A disproportionate number of African Americans, urban and rural, are among those who are poor, unemployed, and who have diminished educational attainment. Statistics indicate that among African Americans living in central cities, 26 percent live below the poverty level compared with 31 percent of those living in rural areas (U.S. Census Bureau, 2001). Unemployment rates among rural and urban African Americans were 12.3% and 13%, respectively, compared to 6% among rural and urban White Americans. Strikingly, over half of rural African Americans have less than 4 years of high school, compared to only about 30 percent of urban African Americans (Allen-Smith, 1995).

Sex is another demographic factor related to depressive symptoms. In general, women are twice as likely to suffer from depressive symptoms as men (Nolen-Hoeksema, 2001). A number of explanations have been offered to account for the higher prevalence of depressive symptoms among women, including biological, psychological, and social factors. In addition, the contribution of women's social roles to depression has received much attention. The role of caring for others has primarily been delegated to women, who at times find themselves simultaneously caring for their children and caring for sick and elderly family members. The inability of women to efficiently and effectively carry out prescribed roles can lead to stress and strain which is oftentimes associated with depression (Piccinelli & Wilkinson, 2000).

Although fulfilling multiple roles is not unique to African American women, it is believed that they are particularly vulnerable to depression related to role strain. African American women have been relied upon as the "pillars of strength, healers, and caretakers of everyone" (Daniel, 1996) often at the expense of their own well being. Further, African American women have carried out these roles with little use of formal services because, historically, racial discrimination and laws prohibited African Americans from benefiting from resources such as adequate health care and educational institutions (Franklin, 1997). Although laws preventing African Americans from acquiring formal services no longer exist, African American cultural beliefs still mandate that the care of family members be undertaken by African American matriarchs (Cochran, Brown, & McGregor, 1999). Thus, many African American women continue to fulfill multiple roles by providing care to children and other dependent family members, while sometimes working outside of the home for pay. These multiple roles may place them at risk for role strain and, subsequently, depression.

OBSTACLES TO DIAGNOSES AND TREATMENT

Although it is estimated that the prevalence of depression among African American women is higher than that among Caucasian women (Kessler et al., 1994), African American women are less likely to voluntarily seek formal treatment for emotional disorders. The low numbers of African Americans seeking formal treatment for emotional disorders has been linked to lack of health insurance, mistrust of the medical community, and the beliefs African Americans hold about depression and other emotional disorders (National Mental Health Association [NMHA], n.d.). According to a survey conducted by the NMHA, only 31 percent of African Americans felt that depression was a medical problem. A majority of African Americans believed depression to be a personal weakness for which prayer and faith alone would serve as treatment.

In addition to obstacles to the diagnoses and treatment of emotional disorders, rural African Americans face obstacles associated with their geographic location. People living in rural communities are often isolated; therefore, they have limited access to formal resources, such as mental health services, and transportation (Holzer, Goldsmith, & Ciarlo, 2000). A large percentage of rural counties lack any mental health services at all (Hartley, Bird, & Dempsey, 1999). For many rural African Americans, access to health care is limited to crisis care, which oftentimes overshadows depressive symptoms (Bushy, 1998). Further, primary care physicians in rural areas may lack the specific mental health training necessary to diagnose depression and emotional disorders (Hartley, Bird, & Dempsey, 1999). Even when rural African Americans are properly diagnosed with emotional disorders, lack of adequate transportation services in rural areas can interfere with ongoing treatment.

CURRENT STUDY

A resource development perspective proposed by Allen and Britt (1983) was used as a theoretical guide in this study to examine and compare emotional health among rural and urban African American women. This perspective suggests that the availability of personal, social, and economic resources should be examined when studying the well being of African American women. In this perspective, personal, social, and economic resources are viewed as three conceptually distinct, but overlapping, resources that can minimize the negative consequences of stressful events. Personal resources are considered to be attributes of the individual, and can include a person's age, health, ease in carrying out roles, and education. Both age and health have been found to negatively correlate with depressive symptoms. Evidence has suggested that as people age there is a decrease in their susceptibility to depression, which may result from increased emotional control or "psychological immunization" to stressful experiences (Jorm, 2000). Depression is also more prevalent among those experiencing physical health problems than among those who are not (Geerlings, Beekman, Deeg, & Van Tilburg, 2000). People who report strain in carrying out their roles have higher levels of depressive symptoms than those who report less strain (Skaff & Pearlin, 1992). It is the inability to effectively and efficiently fulfill multiple social roles that leads to role strain, making one susceptible to depressive symptoms. Fewer depressive symptoms are also found among persons who are more educated (Kessler et al., 2003). Often, educated individuals are exposed less to stressful environments and maintain lifestyles that are conducive to good health.

Social resources encompass primary and secondary relationships which provide sources of social support to individuals. In this particular study, social resources include measures of one's satisfaction with social support, religious practice, family cohesion, and friendships. Individuals who are embedded within social networks that provide them with support often report fewer depressive symptoms than those who are not part of such networks (Saltzman & Holahan, 2002). Likewise familial ties and church affiliations are salient features within African American culture (Hill, 1999) and are expected to positively contribute to their emotional well being. Finally, economic resources such as employment and income refer to the resources that enable persons to fulfill economic needs. Studies have documented the positive relationship among economic resources and emotional health (Lynch, Kaplan, & Shema, 1997).

The current study will examine the role of informal resources, particularly personal, social, and economic resources, on the emotional health of African American women who are caregivers to dependent elderly. The overrepresentation of African Americans in positions associated with depressive symptoms (e.g., low income and low educational status), the higher prevalence rates of depression among women, and the reluctance to seek and obstacles to seeking formal medical treatment for emotional problems put African American women at risk for poor emotional health. Furthermore, because rural African Americans are presented with unique problems associated with the diagnosis and treatment of mental disorders and because they are often overlooked in the mental health literature, this study will compare the roles of informal resources in emotional health among rural and urban dwellers.

Hypotheses

Allen and Britt (1983) posit that personal, social, and economic resources enable African American women to buffer many of the stressors associated with their relatively low social position in American society. Thus, it is hypothesized that both urban and rural African American women who have greater personal, social, and economic resources will be emotionally healthier than those having fewer of these resources. Additionally, it is hypothesized that the effects of personal, social, and economic resources will be greater among rural African American women than among urban African American women because fewer formal resources are available to the former.

Sample and Procedures

The study participants were 261 female caregivers who were providing care to a dependent older adult who had either a functional impairment, defined as an inability to perform two or more basic activities of daily living (Branch, Katz, Kniepmann, & Papsidero, 1984), and/or a cognitive impairment, defined as a score of three or more on the Short Portable Mental Status Questionnaire SPMSQ) (Pfeiffer, 1975). The caregivers in this study were selected from a larger study that examined the structures and outcomes of African American caregivers providing care to dependent elders (Dilworth-Anderson, Williams, & Cooper, 1999). The study participants resided in one of five contiguous counties in the Piedmont region of North Carolina, one urban and four rural. Urban and rural counties were defined using the Federal Office of Management and Budget (OMB) dichotomous classification of metropolitan versus nonmetropolitan counties. With this definition, counties that contain cities with populations of more than 50,000 were considered to be metropolitan counties and all other counties were considered to be nonmetropolitan or rural. In 1990, the urban county in this study contained a city with a population of 181,835 whereas the total populations of the rural counties ranged from 17,265 to 38,892 (U.S. Census Bureau, n.d.). All five counties were classified as Black counties with at least one-third of their populations consisting of African Americans: one rural county was classified as predominantly Black with over half of its population African American (Cromartie, 1999). The final sample consisted of 195 urban and 66 rural dwellers.

Measures

Dependent Variable

Depressive symptoms were measured using a modified version of the Center for Epidemiologic Studies Depression Scale (CES-D; Radloff, 1977). All of the original items on the CES-D were included. However, responses were collapsed to a yes/no format indicating the absence or presence of a symptom in the week prior to the interview. Affirmative responses were given a score of "1" while responses of no were given a score of "0". Responses were summed so that higher scores indicated greater depressive symptoms. With the modified version of the CES-D, scores of 9 or greater are suggestive of clinically significant depressive symptoms (Blazer, Burchett, Service, & George, 1991).

Personal Resources

Age, education, health, and level of role strain were used as measures of personal resources. A dichotomous variable created from those who completed high school or its equivalent and those who did not complete high school was used as a measure of education. Health status was measured using the five-item general health subscale of the RAND Health Survey 1.0, which was adapted from the Medical Outcomes Study (MOS–36) (McHorney, Ware, Lu, & Sherbourne, 1994). Responses from this scale were recoded to percentile scores ranging from 0 to 100 and then averaged with higher scores indicative of better health. A seven-item Global Role Strain Scale developed by Archbold, Stewart, Greenlick, and Harvath (1990) was used to measure the caregiver's level of role strain in carrying out their caregiving duties. Scores on this scale ranged from 7 (no strain) to 28 (maximum strain).

Social Resources

The social resources available to participants were assessed by measuring their satisfaction with social support, religious service attendance, family cohesion, and friendships. The six-item shortened version of the Social Support Questionnaire (SSQ) was used to gauge participant's satisfaction with their social support (Sarason, Sarason, Shearin, & Pierce, 1987). Participants were first asked to give the names of the people they relied upon in each of six areas: to be dependable, to help them to feel relaxed, to accept them, to care about them, to help them to feel better, and to console them. They were then asked to rate how satisfied they were with the support they received in each of the areas. A satisfaction score was derived based on the mean score of the six satisfaction questions and ranged from 1 (least satisfied) to 6 (most satisfied). Religious service attendance was measured with a yes/no response to a question asking participants if they attended a place of worship. The degree of commitment, help, and support family members provided for one another was measured using the Family Cohesion Subscale from the larger Family Environment Scale (Moos, 1974). Scores on this measure ranged from 0 to 9 with higher scores indicating greater family cohesion. Finally, to access the friendships of respondents, they were asked if they had really good friends who were not relatives with whom they spent time.

Economic Resources

The personal income and employment status of participants were used to measure economic resources. Participants were asked to indicate on a chart which income range best described their total personal income during the last year. Responses on the chart were ordered from 1 (less than $10,000) to 10 (more than $50,000) so that higher numbers indicated higher income ranges. Employment status was measured using a dichotomous variable of those who were working either full- or part-time and those who were not working for whatever reason.

Residence in these analyses was defined categorically as either living in a rural county or an urban county. Rural counties were defined as counties containing cities with fewer than 50,000 residents and urban counties contained cities with 50,000 or more residents.

RESULTS

Initial Analyses

Descriptive Statistics

Albeit not statistically significant, the mean CES-D score for the urban women was lower (3.07) than that of the rural women (3.24) (see Table 10.1). Approximately 9 percent of the urban women met the criterion for clinically significant depressive symptoms, whereas

TABLE 10.1   Descriptive Analyses Between Rural and Urban Participants

	Rural (n = 66)		Urban (n = 195)		T
	M	%	M	%	
CES-D	3.24		3.07		.33
Clinical symptoms		14		9	1.15
Age	53.50		54.81		.61
High school diploma		48		69	3.08**
Role strain	12.27		12.84		.93
Health	70.13		72.67		.91
Support satisfaction	5.88		5.86		.30
Attend worship		85		88	.99
Family cohesion	7.02		7.09		.18
Friendships		77		88	2.19*
Income	1.68		2.74		3.86***
Employed		48		58	1.34

Note: A mean income of 1.68 corresponds to an income range of $10,000 to $15,000 per year and 2.74 corresponds to a range of $16,000 to $20,000 per year.
*$p < .05$
**$p < .01$
***$p < .001$

14 percent of the rural women met the criterion. Rural and urban participants were statistically similar in terms of the percentages attending church, and working. They were also similar with regard to age, health, degree of role strain, family cohesion, and satisfaction with social support. The rural and urban participants statistically differed from one another on educational status, friendships, and income. Rural participants were less likely to have a high school diploma and to have nonkin friendships than were urban participants, and also had lower incomes than urban participants.

Pairwise Correlations

Pairwise correlations were conducted for rural and urban participants between the CES-D scores and each of the independent variables (see Table 10.2). Among the rural and urban participants, significant correlations were found between CES-D scores and educational status, health, and role strain (personal resources). Specifi-

TABLE 10.2   Pairwise Correlations Between CES-D Scores and Independent Variables

	Rural (n = 66)	Urban (n = 195)
Personal Resources		
Age	−.002	−.069
High school graduate	−.277*	−.138*
Health	−.537***	−.295***
Role strain	.418***	.421***
Social resources		
Support satisfaction	−.110	−.228**
Attend worship	.076	.016
Family cohesion	−.210†	−.065
Friendships	−.038	−.088
Economic resources		
Income	−.113	−.103
Employed	.031	−.125†

†p < .10
*p < .05
**p < .01
***p < .001

cally, having a high school diploma, good health, and lower levels of role strain were associated with fewer depressive symptoms. Satisfaction with social support (social resources) was negatively related to CES-D scores for urban women only.

Multivariate Analyses

Using the pooled sample of rural and urban participants, multiple regression analyses were conducted first with only main effects and then with interaction effects between residence (urban vs. rural) and each of the independent variables. Residence was not significant in predicting depressive symptoms in the main effects model (see Table 10.3). However, significant main effects were found for all the

TABLE 10.3 Multivariate Regression Predicting Depressive Symptoms (N = 261)

	b	SE	b	SE
Residence (rural vs. urban)	−.08	.24	.35	.54
Age	−.04*	.01	−.04	.02
High school graduation	−1.50**	.48	.73**	.26
Health	−.04***	.01	−.06***	.02
Role strain	.30***	.05	.29***	.06
Support satisfaction	−.79	.58	−.67	.92
Attend worship	1.54*	.63	.52	.35
Family cohesion	−.13	.07	−.14	.10
Friendships	−.56	.56	−.75	.60
Income	−.03	.11	−.13	.22
Working	−.06	.46	−.24	.28
Residence x high school			.09	.26
Residence x health			−.03*	.01
Residence x support			.25	.92
Residence x worship			.39	.35
Residence x cohesion			−.03	.10
Residence x friendships			−.09	.60
Residence x income			−.10	.22
Residence x working			−.54	.28
R^2	.31		.34	

*p < .05
**p < .01
***p < .001

personal resources (age, education, health, and role strain) in the pooled analysis. That is, being older, having a high school diploma, having lower levels of role strain, and having good health were associated with fewer depressive symptoms. Among the social resources, only religious service attendance was predictive of depressive symptoms. Participants who reported that they attended religious services had significantly more depressive symptoms than those who reported that they did not attend religious services. None of the economic resources were significant predictors of depressive symptoms in the pooled analysis. Regarding the interaction model, a significant interaction was found only among residence and health. Although health status was predictive of depressive symptoms for both rural and urban participants, it had a greater impact on depressive symptoms among rural residents.

To address the concern that colinearity among the personal resources and the social and economic resources may have diminished the effect of the social resources by residence interactions, separate interaction models were run in which only the social resources by residence interactions were included in the model (analyses not shown). The results of this analysis did not produce any significant social resources by residence interactions.

DISCUSSION

Using Allen and Britt's (1983) resource development perspective as a guide, the current study examined the roles of personal, social, and economic resources in the emotional health of rural and urban African American women. Findings from this study revealed that depressive symptoms and rates of clinical depressive symptoms did not significantly differ among rural and urban African American women. Partial support was found for the first hypothesis, which stated that having personal, social, and economic resources would have a positive effect on the emotional health of both rural and urban African Americans. Partial support was also found for the second hypothesis that personal, social, and economic resources would be more important in predicting the emotional health of rural African American women than urban African American women.

Pairwise correlations revealed that personal resources were related to depressive symptoms for both groups. Specifically, personal resources such as graduation from high school, limited role strain, and good health were associated with fewer depressive symptoms. These findings are concordant with other research studies which suggest that emotional distress is lower among persons with higher levels of education (Ross, Reynolds, & Geis, 2000), better health (Aro, Nyberg, Absetz, Henriksson, & Loennqvist, 2001) and lower levels of role strain (Beach, Schulz, Yee, & Jackson, 2000). Social resources were correlated with depressive symptoms among urban residents only. Being satisfied with social support was linked to fewer depressive symptoms among urban African American women.

Pooled multiple regression analysis including both rural and urban women indicated that residence was not a significant predictor of depressive symptoms. Instead, all of the personal resources (age, education, health, and role strain) significantly predicted depressive symptoms. Religious attendance was the only social resource that was predictive of depressive symptoms. Rural and urban women who reported that they attended a place of worship had more depressive symptoms than those who reported that they did not attend religious services.

Our second hypothesis posited that personal, social, and economic resources would have a greater impact on rural African American women's emotional health than that of urban African American women. This hypothesis was partially supported when a significant interaction was found among residence and health. The interaction suggested that good health was a stronger predictor of emotional health among rural women than it was among urban women. Poor health may be more of a burden in rural communities because there may be fewer resources available to assist physically compromised persons, such as specialized transportation or support groups. Also, as noted before, many rural African Americans only interface with the medical establishment during crisis situations. Therefore, many rural African Americans may suffer from chronic health problems that go untreated.

IMPLICATIONS AND SUGGESTIONS
FOR FUTURE RESEARCH

The findings from this study have several implications for future studies involving rural African American women and emotional health. First, similar to other studies comparing rural and urban residents (Kessler et al., 2003), this study found that residence was not predictive of depressive symptoms. Instead, this study found that the availability of resources, particularly personal resources, was more predictive of emotional health for African American women than was their rural or urban residence. This finding points to the need for researchers to examine and to understand the lives of rural African Americans. As Conger (1997) has noted, many parts of the rural South, in which rural African Americans are concentrated, are becoming "ghettos" in much the same way as urbanized areas: the young, affluent, and educated leave, which leaves behind the old, poor, and uneducated. The "ghettorization" of rural areas creates social environments that are similar to those found in larger cities. In fact, Conger (1997) points out that rural Southern African Americans are more similar socially to their inner-city counterparts than are those living outside of the larger cities (i.e., the suburbs). The likeness in social environments such as poverty and lowered educational status among rural and urban African Americans can create similar risks to emotional health. Further exploration is needed to understand how differences in the physical environments of rural and urban African Americans affect how they utilize resources to cope with emotional problems.

Second, the finding that poor physical health status is more detrimental to the emotional health of rural African American women than it is for urban women warrants further investigation. An examination and comparison of the types and severity of physical health problems prevalent among rural and urban African Americans may shed light upon this finding. Overall, rural persons suffer from higher incidences of chronic illness and experience more disability and morbidity related to diabetes, cancer, hypertension, heart disease, stroke, and lung disease than their urban counterparts (Mulder et al., 2001). Epidemiological studies show that 25 percent of individuals with a severe chronic medical illness develop depression (Tolman, 1995), making the need to clarify the relationship among physical and emotional health among rural African American women more pertinent.

Finally, counter to other studies (Koenig et al., 1997; Levin & Taylor, 1998), this study found that religious attendance had a positive correlation with depressive symptoms. Rural and urban African

American women who indicated that they attended church had a higher number of depressive symptoms than those who indicated that they did not attend church. It has been suggested that involvement in the church can have positive as well as negative effects (Krause, Ellison, & Wulff, 1998; Nooney & Woodrum, 2002). Church duties can be taxing and exert additional strains on individuals, which may compromise their emotional health. Also, because many African Americans view mental illness as a personal weakness, which prayer and faith can heal (NMHA), it is possible that those experiencing depressive symptoms may be more apt to attend church as a "cure" for emotional problems than those who are not. Future studies are needed to examine the link between church involvement and emotional disorders.

Although the results of this study are important in that they examine resources that are beneficial to the emotional health of African American women and how the importance of these resources differs among rural and urban African American women, several limitations must be noted. The samples of rural and urban African American women used in this study are a small and select group of caregivers to the elderly who are not representative of rural or urban African American women. Thus, caution should be exercised in generalizing the findings of this study to the overall population of rural African American women. It is possible that the unique roles of these women (i.e., caregiving roles) contributed to the lack of differences among them in terms of the use of resources and emotional health. Also, there have been debates over the methods used to determine if a place is rural versus urban. Some researchers argue that dichotomous distinctions between rural and urban that use measures such as population size or density, as were used in this study, do not adequately define or describe the complexities of rural life (Ciarlo & Zelarney, 2000). These authors suggest using alternative ways of defining rural, such as a defining it on a continuum or using measures of the social environment in classifying rural and urban places.

Because we have focused most of our research interests on urban African Americans, there are many unknowns about the lives of rural African Americans. We are not sure how rural African Americans are or will be affected by social problems that were once experienced by only urban persons. Thus, we cannot be sure of the most effective ways to deliver mental health services to the rural

African American population. More research employing different methodologies (e.g., qualitative methods), larger sample sizes, and representative samples are needed to shed light upon rural African American women and emotional health outcomes.

REFERENCES

Allen, L., & Britt, D. W. (1983). Black women in American society: A resource development perspective. *Issues in Mental Health Nursing, 5,* 61–79.

Allen-Smith, J. (1995). Blacks in rural America: Socioeconomic status and policies to enhance the economic well being. In J. B. Stewart & J. E. Allen-Smith (Eds.), *Blacks in rural America.* New Brunswick, NJ: Transaction Publishers.

Archbold, P. G., Stewart, B. J., Greenlick, M. R., & Harvath, T. (1990). Mutuality and preparedness as predictors of caregiver role strain. *Research in Nursing & Health, 13,* 375–384.

Aro, A. R., Nyberg, N., Absetz, P., Henriksson, M., & Loennqvist, J. (2001). Depressive symptoms in middle-aged women are more strongly associated with physical health and social support than with socioeconomic factors. *Nordic Journal of Psychiatry, 55*(3), 191–198.

Beach, S. R., Schulz, R., Yee, J. L., & Jackson, S. (2000). Negative and positive health effects of caring for a disabled spouse: Longitudinal findings from the caregiver health effects study. *Psychology and Aging, 15*(2), 259–271.

Blazer, D., Burchett, B., Service, C., & George, L. K. (1991). The association of age and depression among the elderly: An epidemiologic exploration. *Journal of Gerontology, 46*(6), M210–M215.

Branch, L. G., Katz, S., Kniepmann, K., & Papsidero, J. (1984). A prospective study of functional status among community elders. *American Journal of Public Health, 74*(3), 266–268.

Brown, D. R. (1990). Depression among Blacks: An epidemiologic perspective. In D. Ruiz (Ed.), *Handbook of mental health and mental disorder among Black Americans.* Westport, CT: Greenwood Press.

Bushy, A. (1998). Health issues of women in rural environments: An overview. *Journal of the American Medical Women's Association, 53*(2), 53–56.

Ciarlo, J. A., & Zelarney, P. T. (2000). Focusing on "frontier": Isolated rural America. *Journal of the Washington Academy of Sciences, 86*(3), 1–24.

Cochran, D. L., Brown, D. R., & McGregor, K. C. (1999). Racial differences in the multiple social roles of older women: Implications for depressive symptoms. *The Gerontologist, 39*(4), 465–472.

Conger, R. (1997). The special nature of rural America. *National Institute on Drug Abuse Research Monograph, 168,* 37–52.

Cromartie, J. B. (1999). Minority counties are geographically clustered. [Electronic version]. *Rural conditions and trends, 9*(2), 14–19.

Daniel, R. B. (1996). Allowing illness in order to heal: Sojourning African American women and the AIDS epidemic. In C. F. Collins (Ed.), *African-American women's health and social issues.* Westport, CT: Auburn House.

Dilworth-Anderson, P. (1998). Emotional well being in adult and later life among African Americans: A cultural and sociocultural perspective. In K. W. Schaie & L. Powell (Eds.), *Focus on emotion and adult development: Annual review of gerontology and geriatrics.* New York: Springer Publishing.

Dilworth-Anderson, P., Williams, S. W., & Cooper, T. (1999). Family caregivers to elderly African Americans: caregiver types and structures. *Journal of Gerontology Series B: Psychological Sciences and Social Sciences, 54*(4), S237–S241.

Franklin, D. (1997). *Ensuring inequality: The structural transformation of the African-American.* New York: Oxford University Press.

Geerlings, S. W., Beekman, A. T., Deeg, D. J., & Van Tilburg, W. (2000). Physical illness and the onset and persistence of depression in older adults: An eight-wave prospective community-based study. *Psychological Medicine, 30,* 369–380.

Hartley, D., Bird, D., & Dempsey, P. (1999). Rural mental health and substance abuse. In T. Ricketts (Ed.), *Rural health in the United States* (pp. 159–178). New York: Oxford University Press.

Hill, R. B. (1999). *The strengths of African American families: Twenty-five years later* (2nd ed.). Lanham, MD: University Press of America.

Holzer, C. E., Goldsmith, H. F., & Ciarlo, J. A. (2000). The availability of health and mental health providers by population density. *Journal of the Washington Academy of Sciences, 86*(3), 25–33.

Jorm, A. F. (2000). Does old age reduce the risk of anxiety and depression? A review of epidemiological studies across the adult life span. *Psychological Medicine, 30*(1), 11–22.

Kessler, R. C., Berglund, P., Demler, O., Jin, R., Koretz, D., Merikangas, K. R., Rush, A. J., Walters, E. E., & Wang, P. S. (2003). The epidemiology of major depressive disorder: Results for the National Comorbidity Survey Replication (NCS-R). *Journal of the American Medical Association, 289*(23), 3095–3105.

Kessler, R. C., McGonagle, K. A., Zhao, S., Nelson, C. B., Hughes, H., Eshelman, S., et al. (1994). Lifetime and 12-month prevalence of DSM-III-R psychiatric disorders in the U.S. *Archives of General Psychiatry, 51*(1), 8–19.

Koenig, H. G., Hays, J. C., George, L. K., Blazer, D. G., Larson, D. B., & Landerman, L. R. (1997). Modeling the cross-sectional relationships between religion, physical health, social support, and depressive symptoms. *American Journal of Geriatric Psychiatry, 5*(2), 131–144.

Krause, N., Ellison, C. G., & Wulff, K. M. (1998). Church-based emotional support, negative interaction, and psychological well being: Findings from a national sample of Presbyterians. *Journal of the Scientific Study of Religion, 37,* 725–741.

Levin, J., & Taylor, R. (1998). Panel analyses of religious involvement and well being in African Americans. *Journal for the Scientific Study of Religion, 37,* 695–709.

Lynch, J. W., Kaplan, G. A., & Shema, S. J. (1997). The cumulative impact of sustained economic hardship on physical, cognitive, psychological, and social functioning. *New England Journal of Medicine, 337*(26), 1889–1895.

McHorney, C., Ware, J. E., Lu, R., & Sherbourne, C. D. (1994). The MOS 36-item short-form health survey (SF-36): III. Tests of data quality, scaling assumptions, and reliability across diverse patient groups. *Medical Care, 32*(1), 40–66.

Moos, R. H. (1974). Family environment scale. In R. H. Moos, P. M. Insel, & B. Humphrey (Eds.), *Combined preliminary manual: Family, work, and group environment scales.* Palo Alto, CA: Consulting Psychologists Press.

Mulder, P. L., Kenkel, M. B., Shellenberger, S., Constantine, M. G., Streiegel, R., Sears, S. F., Jr., et al. (2001). *The behavioral health care needs of rural women.* Retrieved August, 19, 2003, from http://www.apa.org/rural/ruralwomen.pdf

National Mental Health Association (n.d.). *Clinical depression and African Americans.* Retrieved September 17, 2002, from http://www.nmha.org/ccd/support/africanamericanfact.cfm

Nolen-Hoeksema, S. (2001). Gender differences in depression. *Current Directions in Psychological Science, 10*(5), 173–176.

Nooney, J., & Woodrum, E. (2002). Religious coping and church-based social support as predictors of mental health outcomes: Testing a conceptual model. *Journal for the Scientific Study of Religion, 41*(2), 359–368.

O'Hare, W. P., & Curry-White, B. (1992). *The rural underclass: Examination of multiple-problem populations in urban and rural settings.* Louisville, KY: Population Reference Bureau, University of Louisville.

Pfeiffer, E. (1975). A short portable mental status questionnaire for the assessment of organic brain deficit in elderly patients. *Journal of the American Geriatrics Society, 23*(10), 433–441.

Piccinelli, M., & Wilkinson, G. (2000). Gender differences in depression: Critical review. *British Journal of Psychiatry, 177*(6), 486–492.

Radloff, L. S. (1977). The CES-D scale: A self-report depression scale for research in the general population. *Applied Psychological Measurement, 1*(3), 385–401.

Ross, C. E., Reynolds, J. R., & Geis, K. J. (2000). The contingent meaning of neighborhood stability for residents' psychological well being. *American Sociological Review, 65*(4), 581–597.

Saltzman, K. M., & Holahan, C. J. (2002). Social support, self-efficacy, and depressive symptoms: An integrative model. *Journal of Social and Clinical Psychology, 21*(3), 309–322.

Sarason, I. G., Sarason, B. R., Shearin, E. N., & Pierce, G. R. (1987). A brief measure of support: Practical and theoretical implications. *Journal of Social and Personal Relationships, 4,* 497–510.

Skaff, M., & Pearlin, L. I. (1992). Caregiving: Role engulfment and the loss of self. *The Gerontologist, 32*(5), 656–664.

Smith, T. S. (1998). Rural rehabilitation: A modern perspective. Arnaudville, LA: Bow River Publishing.

Tolman, A. D. (1995). Major depressive disorder: The latest assessment and treatment strategies. Kansas City, MO: Compact Clinicals.

Wimberly, R., & Morris, L. (1996). *The reference book on regional well being: U.S. regions, the Black Belt, and Appalachia.* Mississippi State, MS: Southern Rural Development Center.

U.S. Census Bureau (n.d.). *North Carolina state data center.* Retrieved September 23, 2002, from http://census.state.nc.us

U.S. Census Bureau (2001). *Current population survey: Annual demographic survey.* Retrieved May 19, 2003, from http://ferret.bls.census.gov/macro/032002/rdcall/2_003.htm

Chapter 11

Effects of Race and Poverty on Perceived Stress Among Rural Women

Janice C. Probst, Charity G. Moore, and Elizabeth G. Baxley

INTRODUCTION

Rural adults, particularly rural women, face unique challenges. Rural adults have less education and lower income than their urban counterparts, are more likely to report food insecurity and hunger, are less likely to have health insurance, and are less likely to see themselves as healthy (Rogers, 1997; Nord, 2002; Schur & Franco, 1999). Professional supports, such as physician services, are less available in rural areas, and the distances from these services are greater (Rosenblatt & Hart, 1999). The potential absence of needed health care is perceived by rural women to be stressful (Hemard, Monroe, Atkinson, & Blalock, 1998). Rural problems are particularly severe among rural minorities, who tend to be concentrated in resource-poor communities (Probst et al., 2002). In this context, rural women, and especially minority and poor women, could be anticipated to experience high levels of stress, with the ensuing effects on health.

Potential stressors have been conceptualized in different typologies. Sheehan (1996) grouped difficult life events and situations into three categories: ecnonomic indicators, lack of social support, and family stress. A second analytic approach groups potential stressors by time: stressor events and chronic hassles (Wijnberg & Reding, 1999). Stressor events are major occurrences that tend to change the ongoing situation, such as the death of a family member, burglary, divorce, loss of a home through disaster or eviction, and similar circumstances as measured, for example, by the Social Readjustment Rating Scale (Holmes & Rahe, 1967). In contrast, chronic hassles represent a continuous, unchangeable situation. Chronic hassles would include economic circumstances, children in the home, chronic illness or physical limitations, and relationship issues (Wijnberg & Reding, 1999).

Both acute and chronic stressors have been shown to be more common among minority women. In a study conducted in Detroit, African American women were much more likely to have experienced acute events, such as personal experience with crime or death of a family member (Williams, 2002). McCallum, Arnold, and Boland (2002), found chronic conditions causing stress to be more characteristic of the lives of poor African Americans. In this population, the most often discussed sources of stress were lack of adequate resources, role-functioning, relationship conflict, and health concerns. Assessment of stressors and stress in rural minority women is difficult to find in the literature. However, qualitative studies suggest that the stressors affecting urban women are also perceived as stressful by rural women, with discrimination as an additional source of stress (Boutain, 2001). Minority women in the U.S. generally have poorer self-reported health status (Hogue, 2002), but have lower levels of access to care as compared with White women. They are more likely to have public, rather than private, health insurance and are more likely to receive care in less than optimal settings such as emergency departments.

The presence of stressors does not necessarily imply that a woman will *experience* stress. While stressor scale values have been linked to biomarkers of stress (Brantley, Deitz, McKnight, Jones, & Tulley, 1988), correlations do not speak to the experience of individuals. A variety of psychological factors are hypothesized to moderate the degree to which adverse events and situations translate into the experience of stress (Williams & Lawler, 2001). The experience of stress, as opposed to the presence of stressors, is not routinely discussed in the literature. A recent study that found no direct relationship between stressors and low birth weight, for example, did not measure experienced stress, which may in part account for the absence of findings (Sheehan, 1998). We were unable to find any large, representative studies of the degree to which rural and minority women experience stress, rather than stressors. The purpose of this study was to explore perceived stress among rural women in a nationally representative sample, with an emphasis on vulnerable populations: low income and minority women. Because the study was exploratory and descriptive, we did not test any theories regarding stress development. We did pose hypotheses regarding the prevalence of stress based on our prior findings in the areas of health services utilization. We anticipated that:

- Stressors such as low income and poor health would be more prevalent among rural women than among urban women, and more prevalent among minority women than white women in each residential category.

- Stressors would be positively related to the experience of stress.

- Rural women would be more likely to report experiencing high stress than urban women, and minority women more likely than White women.

POPULATION STUDIED AND METHODS

We conducted a cross sectional assessment of self-reported stress, using the National Health Interview Survey (NHIS) Adult Prevention Module, 1998 (National Center for Health Statistics 2000). The NHIS is an annual survey conducted for the National Center for Health Statistics by the U.S. Bureau of the Census. It is one of the principal sources of health information on the civilian, noninstitutionalized household population in the United States. The study uses a complex sample design involving multistage sampling and requires use of survey weights for generalization to the U.S. population. The issues we explored were perceived stress, perceived stress effects, and stress reduction activities.

"Rural residence" was defined as living outside a metropolitan statistical area. A metropolitan statistical area consists of a county containing a city of 50,000 or more, plus any adjacent counties that are closely integrated with the central urban area (U.S. Census Bureau, 2003). Race/ethnicity categories were based on an NHIS race/ethnicity composite variable defined as non-Hispanic White, non-Hispanic African American, and Hispanic. Persons of other races were not studied, because the number of rural respondents was too small for accurate analysis. Our analysis was limited to working age women (18–64) resulting in an unweighted sample size of 13,832 women. Population estimates, proportions, standard errors, and co-efficients from multiple logistic regressions were estimated with SAS-callable SUDAAN 8 and SAS 8.1, incorporating survey weight and study design information.

Stress

The NHIS measures stress and stress effects using a four-point Likert scale, asking whether the respondent experienced "a lot of stress, a moderate amount of stress, relatively little stress, or almost no stress at all" during the past 12 months. We defined high stress as the perception of "a lot" of stress, and stress related effects on health as perception of "a lot" of such effects. The NHIS also includes a yes/no question pertaining to steps taken to control or reduce stress in the past year, asking if "any steps to control or reduce the amount of stress" were taken.

Stressors

We examined both recent life events and chronic hassles as potential stressors. Recent life events were defined as a "yes" response to the question, "During the past 12 months, have you had any SERIOUS personal or emotional problems?" Chronic hassles that might cause stress included living in poverty, low education, unmarried marital status, presence of children in the home, self-reported poor health status, limitations in activities of daily living, reporting working in the past week, and lack of health insurance. Poverty was defined as income below $20,000 per year. This is approximately 146% of the Federal poverty level of $13,650 for a family of three in 1998. We did not use actual poverty status, because this value, which requires consideration of various sources of income and family situation, was missing from 20% of all records. Use of the poverty variable could potentially bias our estimates if the variable was nonrandomly missing.

We conducted a multiple logistic regression analysis to determine the factors associated with experiencing "a lot" of stress. These regression models also assessed the associations of race/ethnicity and rural resident status with perceived stress while controlling for the other stressors studied. Associations were determined by odds ratios (OR) and their 95% confidence intervals (95% CI).

POTENTIAL STRESSORS AMONG RURAL AND URBAN WOMEN

The objective disadvantages experienced by rural women are illustrated in Table 11.1. Low income, low education, and poor health are chronic stressors that were more prevalent among rural women of all racial backgrounds. Three of every five African American women and two of every five Hispanic rural women reported a family income under $20,000. Rural white women were also significantly less well off financially than their urban counterparts. One in every eight urban White women had an annual family income of less than $20,000, whereas about one in every four rural White women did so. Rural women overall were more likely to report that they were in fair or poor health than urban women, and less likely to report that they had health insurance. Rural African American women had the highest rates of self-reported poor health. Rural Hispanic women had the highest rates of lack of health insurance, with approximately two of every five rural Hispanic women reporting no health insurance.

Social situations, which can be stressors or supports, were more complex. Hispanic and White rural women were more likely to be married than their urban counterparts. Only a third of African American women, either rural or urban, reported being currently married, suggesting lower social support. At the same time, rural White and African American women were also more likely, whether married or single, to have children in their households, adding mothering as a potential stressor.

Self-reported acute stressors, defined as a serious personal or emotional problems during the past year, were equally distributed.

TABLE 11.1 Characteristics of Rural and Urban Working Age Women, in Percentages, With Standard Errors (SE)

		Total[a] % (SE)	Hispanic % (SE)	White % (SE)	Afr Amer % (SE)
Urban[b]	% race/ethnicity	100.0	12.1	69.4	13.8
	Resources				
	No HS diploma	14.1 (.46)	39.9 (1.2)	8.6 (.48)	19.5 (1.5)
	Worked last week	69.4 (.57)	57.4 (1.3)	71.8 (.68)	68.0 (1.5)
	Income < $20K	19.3 (.50)	35.1 (1.3)	13.1 (.50)	37.6 (1.7)
	Family situation				
	Married	59.5 (.65)	58.2 (1.3)	64.8 (.76)	33.2 (1.5)
	Children in the home	51.0 (.56)	67.6 (1.2)	46.2 (.69)	59.9 (1.4)
	Health				
	Health Status (fair/poor)	8.5 (.29)	12.1 (.77)	6.7 (.33)	14.3 (.83)
	Limitations in activities	11.0 (.36)	9.1 (.67)	10.7 (.44)	14.0 (.89)
	Insurance (none)	14.8 (.42)	35.2 (1.3)	10.2 (.44)	20.1 (1.2)
Rural[b]	% race/ethnicity	100.0	4.3	84.5	8.8
	Resources				
	No HS diploma	16.1 (.81)	39.8 (3.7)	13.7 (.81)	28.3 (3.0)
	Worked last week	67.3 (1.1)	54.5 (4.5)	68.9 (1.2)	58.9 (3.2)
	Income < $20K	26.6 (1.2)	41.7 (4.6)	22.5 (1.2)	58.5 (3.8)
	Family situation				
	Married	66.9 (1.2)	65.5 (3.1)	70.3 (1.3)	34.1 (3.1)
	Children in the home	51.0 (1.0)	62.1 (4.1)	48.7 (1.2)	64.5 (2.7)
	Health, rural women				
	Health Status (poor)	11.9 (.62)	17.9 (3.1)	10.7 (.62)	21.1 (2.5)
	Limitations in activities	14.4 (.76)	10.7 (2.1)	14.3 (.81)	16.9 (2.3)
	Insurance (none)	17.7 (.88)	39.3 (6.1)	15.3 (.99)	30.1 (3.5)

[a]Total includes "Other" race. Sum of percentages for Hispanic, White, and African American does not equal 100 for this reason.
[b]All race comparisons within a residence category are significant at p < .001 or better, with one exception. For rural women, race/ethnicity differences in the proportion of women reporting limitations in activities were not statistically significant (p = .1569).
[c]P-values for rural-urban comparisons within race/ethnicity groups are as follows:

	Total	Hispanic	White	Black
No HS diploma	0.0289	0.988	< 0.0001	0.0089
Work	0.0914	0.5487	0.0297	0.0076
Income	< 0.0001	0.1770	< 0.0001	< 0.0001
Married	< 0.0001	0.0470	0.0001	0.7958
Children	0.8579	0.1830	0.0706	0.1298
Health	< 0.0001	0.0664	< 0.0001	0.0198
Limitations	0.0001	0.4873	0.0002	0.2465
Insurance	0.0044	0.5261	< 0.0001	0.0065

Approximately 16 percent of women, both urban and rural and regardless of race/ethnicity, reported such problems.

REPORTED STRESS

Prevalence of Stress

Although chronic stressors such as low income and poor health status were more prevalent in rural areas and among minorities, the perceived prevalence of stress was slightly less among rural women than urban women (Table 11.2). This effect held true across racial groups. For example, 22 percent of urban African American women and only 19 percent of rural African American women reported experiencing "a lot" of stress.

Racial differences among women who reported *high* levels of stress were more consistent than rural-urban differences. In both

TABLE 11.2   Reported Levels of Stress and Stress Effects, by Residence and Race/Ethnicity, in Percentages, With Standard Errors (SE)

	Total % (SE)	Hispanic % (SE)	White % (SE)	Afr Amer % (SE)
Urban *Reported stress:*				
A lot	26.2 (.54)	20.7 (1.1)	28.0 (.64)	21.7 (1.4)
Moderate	38.5 (.59)	28.5 (1.1)	41.6 (.70)	31.3 (1.4)
Little	21.2 (.48)	24.4 (1.1)	20.0 (.59)	24.7 (1.3)
Almost none	14.2 (.44)	26.5 (1.1)	10.5 (.47)	22.3 (1.4)
Rural *Reported stress:*				
A lot	24.9 (1.0)	19.8 (2.7)	25.8 (1.1)	18.5 (2.9)
Moderate	36.5 (.98)	30.9 (3.7)	37.6 (1.1)	28.3 (3.2)
Little	24.5 (1.0)	27.6 (3.6)	23.8 (1.1)	30.0 (3.2)
Almost none	14.1 (.90)	21.8 (2.6)	12.8 (.95)	23.1 (3.7)

Race effects:
   Within urban: p < .0001
   Within rural: p = .0005
Urban-Rural effects:
Total: p = .0257
   Within Hispanic: p = .1966
   Within White: p < .0001
   Within Black: p = .3468

urban and rural areas, White women were more likely to report "a lot" of stress than were their African American and Hispanic counterparts. This is notable in that it occurred despite the greater prevalence of chronic life difficulties in minority populations. While one in four (25.8%) rural White women reported experiencing a lot of stress, this proportion drops to one in five (19.8% and 18.5%) for rural minority women. Conversely, minority women were much more likely to report experiencing "little" or "almost no" stress.

While it is possible that minority women interpret "stress" differently, this appears unlikely. Among rural women, those reporting "a lot" of stress were generally more likely to experience a particular stressor (Table 11.3). For example, nearly a third of high-stress women, versus a quarter of lower-stress women, had low income. Similarly, more than one in five women reporting high stress also reported poor to fair health, versus just less than one in 10 women who reported lower stress levels. This relationship was most noticeable for recent life events. Among women who perceived themselves under a lot of stress, 40.4 percent had experienced a "serious personal/emotional" problem in the past year, versus only 7.8 percent among women with less stress.

Examining Stress Among All U.S. Women Age 18 to 64 Years

Holding all things equal through multiple logistic regression, the factor most strongly associated with perceived high stress was the experience of serious personal/emotional problems within the past year (Table 11.4). Women who reported the presence of serious personal or emotional problems had more than seven times the odds of reporting high levels of stress than women who did not report serious problems. Health-related chronic stressors and age had the next highest associations with perceived stress. Women in self-reported poor or fair health were more likely to report high stress than healthier women, and women who reported experiencing limits in their ability to work or participate in normal activities were more likely to report high stress than their counterparts without such limits. Interestingly, lack of health care coverage was not a significant contributor to the risk of stress, despite perception of

TABLE 11.3 Distribution of Demographic and Need Variables, by Level of Stress, in Percentages, With Standard Errors (SE)

	A lot of stress % (SE)	Moderate to almost none % (SE)
Number of rural women (weighted population estimate)	4,165,628	12,584,070
Race/ethnicity		
Hispanic	3.4% (.52)	4.6% (0.81)
White	89.9% (1.2)	85.8% (1.3)
Black	6.6% (1.2)	9.6% (1.1)
Age categories		
18–24	15.4% (1.7)	14.7% (1.0)
25–40	38.2% (2.0)	37.7% (1.3)
41–55	34.3% (2.2)	32.5% (1.3)
56–64	12.1% (1.6)	15.2% (0.9)
Region		
Northeast	14.1% (1.5)	9.7% (1.2)
Midwest	30.3% (2.6)	32.4% (1.6)
South	42.6% (3.0)	45.7% (1.9)
West	13.1% (1.2)	12.1% (1.3)
Education		
No HS diploma	18.5% (1.9)	15.2% (0.8)
High school or better	81.5% (1.9)	84.8% (0.8)
Employment status		
Working last week	64.4% (2.1)	68.3% (1.3)
Not working last week	35.6% (2.1)	31.7% (1.3)
Income		
Below $20K	32.5% (2.2)	24.6% (1.3)
$20K or more	67.5% (2.2)	75.4% (1.3)
Family Situation		
Married, no children	29.6% (1.9)	32.1% (1.0)
Married, children	32.3% (2.1)	36.6% (1.2)
Not Married, no children	20.1% (1.6)	17.4% (1.1)
Not Married, children	18.1% (1.6)	13.9% (0.8)
Self-reported health status		
Poor to fair	21.3% (1.8)	9.1% (0.7)
Good to excellent	78.7% (1.8)	90.9% (0.7)
Limitations in IADL		
Limited	23.8% (1.7)	11.4% (0.8)
Not limited	76.2% (1.7)	88.6% (0.8)
Health insurance		
Uninsured	18.3% (1.7)	17.4% (1.0)
Insured	81.7% (1.7)	82.6% (1.0)
Serious personal/emotional problem in past 12 months		
Yes	40.4% (2.2)	7.8% (0.6)
No	59.6% (2.2)	92.2% (0.6)

TABLE 11.4 Factors Associated With the Odds That a Woman Will Report "a Lot" of Stress During the Past Twelve Months*

Variable	Odds Ratio	Lower 95%	Upper 95%
Living in an urban area	1.19	1.02	1.37
Minority race and family income:			
Hispanic, less than $20,000/year	0.56	0.42	0.75
Non Hispanic White, less than $20,000/year	1.37	1.17	1.61
Non Hispanic AA, less than $20,000/year	0.56	0.42	0.76
Hispanic, more than $20,000/year	0.63	0.51	0.77
Non Hispanic AA, more than $20,000/year	0.66	0.53	0.85
Non Hispanic White, more than $20,000/year	1.00	–	–
No health insurance coverage	1.11	0.96	1.28
Limited in IADLs	1.79	1.48	2.16
Self-reported fair or poor health	1.92	1.58	2.33
Serious personal/emotional problems in past year	7.63	6.76	8.62
Family situation, comp to married, no children			
Married with child(ren)	1.01	0.86	1.17
Not married, no child(ren)	1.18	1.01	1.38
Not married, child(ren)	1.20	0.99	1.44
Working versus not working	1.28	1.14	1.44
Compared to ages 56–64: 18–24	1.88	1.52	2.33
25–40	1.91	1.60	2.27
41–55	1.54	1.27	1.87

*Multiple logistic regression analysis. Race, income, and the race/income interaction effect were each significant. To facilitate interpretation of findings, main and interaction effects for race and income have been calculated and expressed for each category. Two nonsignificant effects are not shown. These are region of the country and education (high school graduate versus less education).

poor health and limitations, after other characteristics of the woman's situation were held equal.

Day-to-day hassles were also associated with stress. Low-income women were more likely to report high stress than women whose family income was greater than $20,000 per year. Women who were working outside the home were more likely to report high stress than other women. Family situation, defined as one of four possible combinations of marital status and presence/absence of children in the home, showed a tendency for increasing stress among persons who were not currently married when compared with married women without children. Younger women were more likely to report high stress than women aged 56–64 years. Education had no relationship with reported stress. This was surprising, as we had assumed that low education, because of its implications for resources (low income, lack of health insurance) and coping skills, would be associated with increased stress. The close correlation between education and eventual resources may serve to mask the economic effects of education. It is also possible that coping skills are acquired outside of formal education. Region was also not a significant factor when examining stress across the whole population.

The key independent variables were rural residence, race, and income. After controlling for potential stressors, rural women in general had *lower* odds of experiencing high stress than urban women. Similarly, racial minorities had lower odds of reporting high stress than White women. Further, minority race had a protective effect for low-income women, as indicated by the significant interaction term. While low income increased the odds that a woman would report high stress, among minority women nationally this increase was less than among White women.

Race and Poverty Effects: Stress Among Rural Women

When multiple logistic regression analysis was used to explore high stress within *rural* women, the patterns were similar to those observed among all women. Recent events, characterized as serious personal or emotional problems in the past year, were most closely associated with self-reported high stress. Rural women who reported such experiences were more likely to report high stress compared with rural women not reporting recent problems (Table 11.5). Health related issues, such as perceived fair or poor health and the experience of limitations in activities of daily living, were the next highest source of risk for stress. Age effects were also similar among rural and urban women, with the odds of reported stress declining with age.

TABLE 11.5 Factors Associated With the Odds That a Rural Woman Will Report "a Lot" of Stress During the Past Twelve Months.*

Variable	Odds Ratio	Low 95%	Upper 95%
Minority race			
Hispanic	0.56	0.37	0.87
African American	0.58	0.38	0.87
Compared to the NE:			
Midwest	0.69	0.50	0.95
South	0.66	0.48	0.89
West	0.77	0.57	1.04
Family income less than $20,000/year	1.19	0.90	1.57
No health care coverage	0.94	0.70	1.26
Limited in any way in IADLs	1.48	1.02	2.15
Self-reports fair or poor health	1.86	1.19	2.91
Serious personal/emotional problems in past year	7.29	5.37	9.90
Compared to married, no children:			
Mar w/children	0.91	0.67	1.25
Single no children	0.93	0.65	1.31
Single w/children	1.00	0.64	1.55
Employed outside the home	1.20	0.89	1.61
Compared to ages 56–64:			
18–24	1.69	1.10	2.60
25–40	1.66	1.16	2.38
41–55	1.36	0.90	2.04

*Multiple logistic regression analysis. Nonsignificant effects of education (high school graduate versus less) are not shown.

Employment outside the home, which was associated with a higher risk of stress among all women, had a similar association among rural women, but the effect was not significant. The same was true for being single, with or without children. As was the case among all women, lack of health insurance was not statistically significant after controlling for other situations in the person's life.

Regional effects, not found for the nation as a whole, emerged when analyzing perceived stress in rural women. Compared with women living in the Northeast, rural women living in the Midwest and South were less likely to report high stress. Living in the West also tended to be protective, but the effects did not reach statistical significance.

The key independent variables of race and low income status had effects among rural women similar to those found among all women. Minority race continued to be associated with lower odds of reporting high stress: rural Hispanic and African American women were less likely to report high stress than were rural White women. Lower income was positively, but not significantly, associated with reporting "a lot" of stress among rural women. Because low income was not significant, there were no significant interaction effects; minority race/ethnicity did not modify the risk of stress associated with low income.

Perceived Effects of Stress on Health and Prevalence of Stress Reduction Activities Among Women Reporting "a Lot" of Stress

Among non-Hispanic White women reporting "a lot" of stress in the past 12 months, about three of every four, regardless of rural/urban residence, reported experiencing "a lot" or "some" of effects of stress on health (Table 11.6). Urban minority women reported more stress effects on health than their rural counterparts. White women reported participating in stress reduction activities more than any other group (68.3%), followed by African Americans (64.7%) and Hispanics (56.40%). Among White and African American women, stress reduction activities were more commonly reported by urban residents. The situation was reversed among Hispanics, with more rural-dwelling Hispanics involved in stress-reduction activities.

DISCUSSION

Stressors have been categorized by different authors as chronic hassles or major life events. How these categories of stressors are translated into actual perceived stress has been studied less often. This study sought to explore the effects of urban and rural residence, race and low income on experienced stress.

Externally defined stressors, as anticipated in our first hypothesis, were more common among rural than among urban women, and particularly among minority women. Levels of objectively defined difficulty among rural women were almost startling: nearly three in

TABLE 11.6 Women Reporting "a Lot" of Stress in Past Twelve Months Who Also Report Stress Reduction Activities and Effects of Stress on Health, in Percentages, With Standard Error (SE)

	Rural % (SE)	Urban % (SE)
Stress reduction activities		
Total	63.9 (1.9)	67.7 (1.0)
Hispanic	63.2 (8.4)	55.8 (2.9)
Non Hispanic White	65.3 (1.9)	69.2 (1.2)
Non Hispanic AA	45.0 (6.3)	67.6 (3.0)
Reporting "a lot" or "some" effects on health		
Total	76.3 (1.9)	77.0 (.95)
Hispanic	76.1 (5.8)	84.5 (1.8)
Non Hispanic White	77.1 (2.1)	75.9 (1.2)
Non Hispanic AA	64.9 (6.0)	78.3 (2.3)

p-values for comparisons of stress reduction activities and effects on health:
Race effect for stress reduction activities:
    Within Urban: $p = .0004$
    Within Rural: $p = .0342$
Race effect for stress effects on health:
    Within Urban: $p = .0007$
    Within Rural: $p = .1878$
Rural/urban effect for stress reduction activities: Total: $p = .0716$
    Within Hispanic: $p = .4258$
    Within White: $p = .0848$
    Within Black: $p = .0070$
Rural/urban effect for stress effects on health: Total: $p = .7157$
    Within Hispanic: $p = .1767$
    Within White: $p = .6118$
    Within Black: $p = .0424$

every five rural African American women, and about two in every five rural Hispanic women, had a family income that was less than $20,000 per year. Possibly contributing to low income, rural women, with the exception of Hispanic women, were less likely to be employed, and more likely to report poor to fair health status. On the other hand, rural women, with the exception of African Americans, were more likely to be married than their urban peers, so social support from a spouse may be a source of resilience.

As anticipated in our second hypothesis, all women were at higher risk of *experiencing stress* when they reported poor health or limitations in activities, had low incomes, or had children but not a partner. Surprisingly, our third hypothesis, that greater stress would be reported by rural women and particularly minority rural women, was not supported. The prevalence of experienced stress was lower among rural women and minority women than among their urban, White counterparts. African American and Hispanic women in rural and urban areas, who had quantifiably more life difficulties, were less likely to report high stress than White women. Further, when assessed at the national level, minority status seemed to buffer the effects of low income on reported stress. Participation in stress reduction activities by women reporting high stress yielded similar findings, with White women reporting such activities more often.

When the analysis focused on rural women, similar results were found. Rural minority women, with sociodemographic and need factors held constant, were less likely to report high stress than rural White women. Further, interesting regional effects emerged among rural populations, with residence in the South or Midwest being less stressful than residence in the Northeast, all considerations equal. This suggests that findings among rural minorities, who tend to be geographically concentrated in the South and West, are not a function of local culture. Both regional and minority rural cultures may have protective effects for reported stress.

Our findings raise far more questions than they answer. A profitable approach to future research into experienced stress might be to explore unique sources of support and resilience in rural areas. Studies conducted in Britain (Paykel, Abbott, Jenkins, Brugha, & Meltzer, 2000) and Australia (Brown, Young, & Byles, 1999) found lower stress in rural women. Additional work on rural American women, perhaps using more sensitive definitions of rurality such as the Rural Urban Continuum Codes, could help specify the types of rural community offering the lowest stress profile. Similarly, perhaps research into minority women should move its focus from their demographic disadvantages to their unique strengths.

Lower levels of perceived stress among minority women may have positive or negative origins. From a negative perspective, response to stressors may be internalized, with adverse effects on health (Hogue, 2002). This "weathering hypothesis" characterizes poorer health among minority women as a consequence of the health effects of internalized racism and unacknowledged, suppressed stress. For example, African American women who report greater experience with personal discrimination have poorer self-reported health (Schulz et al., 2000). Additional research is needed to examine relationships among experienced stressors, perceived stress, somatization, and health status within minority populations.

A more positive explanation of lower stress among minority women is offered by "John Henryism" and other concepts of hardiness (Williams & Lawler, 2001). John Henry, the "steel drivin' man" of the song, was willing to pit himself against a steam engine. Rural minority women, with lower (and perhaps more realistic) assessments of the support available to them, may perceive adverse events as a challenge to be overcome, rather than mourned. When asked to indicate their source of support, African American women were most likely to credit "God," while White women indicated that their spouse was the source of support (Bourjolly & Hirschman, 2001). The lower prevalence of depression, a correlate to perceived stress, among African American than White adults has been hypothesized to be related to a higher prevalence of strong spiritual faith in the African American community (Williams, 2000).

Spiritual support assumes that the respondent will herself take action in the physical world. If spiritual strength, hardiness, and other factors empower minority women to handle potentially stressful circumstances more effectively than White women, the next question becomes how these characteristics are developed, and how effective programs might be designed to promote hardiness in minority communities (Hogue, 2002).

Our study, while taking the positive step of not confusing stressors with stress, nonetheless contains several limitations. First, the definition of "rural" used by NHIS was based on the metropolitan/nonmetropolitan definition. Residents of rural counties that support large towns may have much different experiences than residents of low-density counties with few settlement areas. Similarly, analysis that used the Rural-Urban Commuting Area classification of counties might have revealed differences among places of residence based on both size and links to larger urban areas. Second, the measures of stressors and stress were brief. However, the somewhat simple measure of stress did correlate with the presence of stressors, as defined by the literature, in a woman's life. Future work into stress and stressors and health should consider exploring national data sets, such as the NHIS.

Finally, the NHIS, like most national surveys conducted under the auspices of the National Center for Health Statistics, oversamples minority populations but does not oversample rural populations nor, in particular, rural minorities. Since the rural population is proportionately more "White" than the urban population, the absence of rural oversampling results in very small numbers for minority populations. The actual number of rural women surveyed in 1998 was greatest among White women (2,015), followed by African American women (297), and Hispanics (262). Analyses for persons of "other" race—in rural areas, principally Native Americans—could not be performed because there were too few observations (68) for valid projection.

CONCLUSION

We cannot assume that all women react similarly to the presence of stressors. Despite objective measures of more stressors, rural women perceived less stress than their urban counterparts. The same was true when comparing across race/ethnicity groups. White women perceived higher levels of stress, regardless of location of residence, than did minority women, despite the fact that minority women experienced a greater number of life difficulties. We hypothesize that hardiness and varying cultural expectations affect perceived stress. Future studies, particularly using longitudinal designs with adequate representation of rural and minority women, should explore sources of resiliency in this population.

REFERENCES

Bourjolly, J. N., & Hirschman, K. B. (2001). Similarities in coping strategies but differences in sources of support among African-American and White women coping with breast cancer. *Journal of Psychosocial Oncology, 19*(2), 17–38.

Boutain, D. M. (2001). Discourses of worry, stress, and high blood pressure in rural south Louisiana. *Journal of Nursing Scholarship, 33*(3), 225–230.

Brantley, P. J., Dietz, L. S., McKnight, G. T., Jones, G. N., & Tulley, R. (1988). Convergence between the Daily Stress Inventory and endocrine measures of stress. *Journal of Consulting and Clinical Psychology, 56*(4), 549–551.

Brown, W. J., Young, A. F., & Byles, J. E. (1999). Tyranny of distance? The health of mid-age women living in five geographical areas of Australia. *Australian Journal of Rural Health, 7*(3), 148–154.

Hemard, J. B., Monroe, P. A., Atkinson, E. S., & Blalock, L. B. (1998). Rural women's satisfaction & stress as family health care gatekeepers. *Women and Health, 28*(2), 55–77.

Hogue, C. J. R. (2002). Toward a systematic approach to understanding—and ultimately eliminating—African American women's health disparities. *Women's Health Issues, 12*(5), 222–237.

Holmes, T. H., & Rahe, R. H. (1967). The Social Readjustment Rating Scale. *Journal of Psychosomatic Research, 11*, 213–218.

McCallum, D. M., Arnold, S. E., & Bolland, J. M. (2002). Low-income African-American women talk about stress. *Journal of Social Distress and the Homeless, 11*(3), 249–263.

National Center for Health Statistics (2000). Data File Documentation, National Health Interview Survey, 1998. Hyattsville, MD: Author.

Nord, M. (2002). Rates of food insecurity and hunger unchanged in rural households. *Rural America, 16*(4), 42–47.

Paykel, E. S., Abbott, R., Jenkins, R., Brugha, T. S., & Meltzer, H. (2000). Urban-rural mental health differences in Great Britain: Findings from the national morbidity survey. *Psychological Medicine, 30*(2), 269–280.

Probst, J. C., Samuels, M. E., Jespersen, K. P., Willert, K., Swann, R. S., & McDuffie, J. A. (2002). *Minorities in Rural America: An Overview of Population Characteristics (Grant No. 6 U1C RH 00045-01)*. Rockville, MD: Federal Office of Rural Health Policy, Health Resources and Services Administration.

Rogers, C. C. (1997). *Changes In The Social And Economic Status Of Women By Metro-Nonmetro Residence.* Economic Research Service, U.S. Department of Agriculture, Agriculture Information, Bulletin No. 732.

Rosenblatt, R. A., & Hart, L. G. (1999). Physicians and rural America. In T. C. Ricketts, III (Ed.), *Rural health in the United States.* New York: Oxford University Press.

Schulz, A., Israel, B., Williams, D., Parker, E., Becker, A., & James, S. (2000). Social inequalities, stressors and self reported health status among African American and White women in the Detroit metropolitan area. *Social Science & Medicine 51*, 1639–1653.

Schur, C. L., & Franco, S. J. (1999). Access to health care. In T. C. Ricketts, III (Ed.), *Rural health in the United States.* New York: Oxford University Press.

Sheehan, T. J. (1996). Creating a psychosocial measurement model from stressful life events. *Social Science & Medicine, 43*(2), 265–271.

Sheehan, T. J. (1998). Stress and low birth weight: A structural modeling approach using real life stressors. *Social Science and Medicine, 47*(10), 1503–1512.

U.S. Census Bureau (2003). About Metropolitan and Micropolitan Statistical Areas. Retrieved June 30, 2003, from http://www.census.gov/population/www/estimates/aboutmetro.html

Wijnberg, M. H., & Reding, K. M. (1999). Reclaiming a stress focus: The hassles of rural, poor single mothers. *Families in Society, 80*(5), 506–515.

Williams, D. R. (2000). Race, stress and mental health. In C. J. R. Hogue, M. A. Hargraves, & K. S. Colins (Eds.), *Minority health in America: Findings and policy implications from the Commonwealth Fund Minority Health Survey.* Baltimore, MD: Johns Hopkins University Press.

Williams, D. R. (2002). Racial/ethnic variations in women's health: The social imbeddedness of health. *American Journal of Public Health, 92*(4), 588–597.

Williams, D., & Lawler, K. A. (2001). Stress and illness in low-income women: The roles of hardiness, John Henryism, and race. *Women and Health, 32*(4), 61–75.

Chapter 12

Evaluation of Nutrition Education and Exercise in a Health Promotion and Wellness Program for Older Adults

Cathy B. Parrett

In 1998, 20% of the United States population lived in rural or nonmetropolitan counties (Eberhardt et al., 2001). This percentage has decreased since 1920 when 49 percent of the U.S. population lived in rural areas (U.S. Congress, Office of Technology Assessment, 1990). Approximately 15 percent of the rural population in the U.S. is 65 years old or older compared with 12 percent in urban areas. (Rosenthal & Fox, 2000). Rural elderly are usually female, more likely to be poor, and less educated (Eberhardt et al., 2001; Ormond, Wallin, & Goldenson, 2000).

Advancing age predisposes individuals to chronic age-related disorders and the attendant disabilities. In addition, these disorders and the associated disabilities make aging difficult and pose a significant challenge to our health care system (Cassel, 2001) especially in rural settings where provider shortages may be present or transportation constraints may limit access to health care (Rosenthal & Fox, 2000). Limitations with activities such as mobility and self-care increase with age (Administration on Aging, 2001). The rural elderly have higher rates of limitation than urban elderly; 18 percent compared with 12 percent for men and 19 percent compared with 14 percent for women (Eberhardt et al., 2001). Mainous and Kohrs (1995) reported that 42.3 percent of 1000 rural elderly surveyed had difficulty performing activities of daily living such as bathing and instrumental activities such as shopping. In addition, almost 12 percent had depressive symptoms. These limitations threaten the ability of the older adult to function successfully in the community. Maintaining independence is a concern for both urban and rural older adults and is dependent upon the level of mental and physical functioning (Johnson, 1991).

Butler (1995) suggests that disease and dysfunction can be postponed through prevention. Further, he argues that prevention is essential to reduce the social and economic costs of disease. At the national level, *Healthy People 2010* builds upon past initiatives that recognized the prevention of functional decline and preservation of independence as priorities for health care of older adults (U.S. Department of Health and Human Services [USDHHS], 2000). However, goals for improving the health of the nation's residents through health promotion and disease prevention can be achieved only if rural populations are included (Agency for Health Care Policy and Research [AHCPR], 1996). *Rural Healthy People 2010*, a companion document to *Healthy People 2010*, discusses rural health concerns and describes models of practice that could lead to improved access to health care and quality of life (Gamm, Hutchison, Dabney, & Dorsey, 2003).

Components of successful aging, as defined by Rowe and Kahn (1997) include (1) low probability of disease and disease-related disability, (2) active engagement with life, and (3) high cognitive and physical capacity.

LOW PROBABILITY OF DISEASE AND DISEASE-RELATED DISABILITY

This component refers not only to the absence or presence of a disease process but also the absence, presence, or severity of risk factors (Rowe & Kahn, 1997). Research exploring the role of macro-nutrients may reduce risk factors associated with chronic disease (McCarron et al., 1997). Therefore, primary and secondary preventive health interventions such as educational opportunities, immunizations, and health screening promote the process of successful aging (Saunders, 1999).

ACTIVE ENGAGEMENT WITH LIFE

The second component of successful aging is active engagement with life, which includes maintaining relationships with other people and performing activities that are productive (Rowe & Kahn, 1997). Links between social support and health include: (a) lack of social ties or isolation influence health; (b) social support has a direct positive effect on health; (c) social support can buffer health related effects of aging; and (d) no single type of social support is uniformly effective for all people (Seeman et al., 1995). Additionally, disorders associated with mental functioning, such as depression, influence productive activities and fulfilling relationships. Consequently, successful engagement in life is affected (USDHHS, 2000).

MAXIMIZING COGNITIVE AND
PHYSICAL FUNCTION

Successful aging depends, among other factors, on maintaining a level of cognitive ability that allows a person to interact with the environment in an appropriate and effective manner (Teri, McCurry, & Logsdon, 1997). Factors associated with "high mental function" include education, being physically active, having good lung function and high "self-efficacy" (Berkman et al., 1993).

Reduction in the capacity to perform common physical functions may prevent participation in productive and recreational activities. Both sociodemographic and health status characteristics affect physical performance. More specifically, being older, having an income of less than $10,000 per year, higher body mass, high blood pressure, depressive symptoms, and lower cognitive performance were predictive of declines in physical performance or ability (Bruce,

Seeman, Merrill, & Blazer, 1994; Seeman et al., 1994). Behavioral predictors of maintaining physical performance include leisure activity, emotional support from friends, and moderate levels of exercise activity (Rowe & Kahn, 1997).

Rowe and Kahn (1998) assert that it is never too late to begin healthy habits such as cessation of smoking, eating nutritious foods, and exercising. More important, it is never too late to benefit from these changes. Health promotion and wellness programs have suggested improvements in health for older adults (King et al., 2000; List, Maskay, Blumberg, & Banik, 1999; Shellman, 2000; Wallace et al., 1998).

The purpose of this project was to evaluate the effect of nutrition education and exercise interventions on nutritional risk, depression, and physical performance in a health promotion and wellness program at a government-subsidized housing facility. More specifically, the study sought to address the following questions: (1) Does a nutrition education intervention reduce nutritional risk for senior adults? (2) Do exercise and movement interventions (walking or chair exercises) improve physical performance of senior adults? (3) Do exercise and movement interventions (walking or chair exercises) reduce depressive symptoms of senior adults?

PROGRAM DESCRIPTION

The Wellness in Senior Housing (WISH) model is a program designed to enhance the quality of living for senior adults in housing communities (Koch, 2001). This holistic wellness and health promotion program is designed to encourage healthy lifestyle choices by the older adult and to encourage seeking health care options early through appropriate referrals.

Components of the program include health education, physical education and activity, nutrition education, health services referral, behavioral health education and referral, healthy and safe senior environment, spiritual support, and social and community support. The program incorporates principles of Bandura's social cognitive theory, including self-efficacy. Goals of the program are to: (1) encourage healthy lifestyle choices by older adults living in senior housing; (2) encourage seniors to seek health care options early through appropriate referral; (3) incorporate holistic health care by addressing mind, body, and spirit in program activities; (4) invite additional community agencies to join in collaborative efforts to sustain wellness programming in senior housing, thereby maximizing resource utilization and minimizing duplication efforts: and (5) promote measurable, sustainable health benefits for senior participants.

METHODS

Study Design

This descriptive-correlational study employed a quasi-experimental design with one-group pretest-posttest assessment to evaluate nutritional status, mood, and physical function.

The Setting

This study was conducted in a government subsidized apartment facility designed for senior adults which was located in the southeastern United States. To be eligible for this housing arrangement, older adults must meet specific income criteria. At the time of the evaluation, the population of the apartment community included 85 percent ($n = 40$) women and 15 percent ($n = 7$) men. Residents had an average age of 72 and an average income of $785 per month.

Sample

A convenience sample that included 57 percent (n = 27 of 47) of the total resident population was used in the research activity. Inclusion criteria specified that participants be 62 years of age or older, a resident of the housing facility, have the ability to understand and follow instructions, the ability to communicate in English, be cognitively intact, and physically capable of participation in exercise interventions.

Participants ranged in age from 63 to 89 years ($M = 74.11$, $SD = 6.39$). Years of education ranged from 5 to 20 years ($M = 11.78$, $SD = 3.52$). Ninety-three percent were women and seven percent were men. Most of the individuals had lived most of their life in a rural environment. Further, the sample included White (81%), Black (15%), and Hispanic (4%) participants. Baseline data indicated that 56 percent ($n = 15$) of the sample participated in an exercise activity three times per week for at least 30 minutes prior to the study.

Most participants reported at least one chronic condition after being asked if a health care provider had told them that they had any of these conditions. The conditions that were reported most often were high blood pressure ($n = 18$), arthritis ($n = 18$), diabetes ($n = 10$), heart attack ($n = 7$), cancer ($n = 7$), stroke ($n = 3$), and hip fracture ($n = 3$). There were no changes in these frequencies at post-test.

The attrition rate was 11 percent (3 of 27). In general, the individuals who dropped out of the study had more chronic conditions, longer timed walk scores, and higher depression scores at pretest. Most of those who dropped out of the study also stated they did not feel like completing the post-test forms.

Instruments

Nutritional risk was measured using the DETERMINE Your Nutritional Health (DETERMINE) Checklist (Nutrition Screening Initiative, 1992). The Nutrition Screening Initiative was a project of the American Academy of Family Physicians, The American Dietetic Association, and the National Council on the Aging, Inc., and was funded, in part, by a grant from the Ross Products Division, Abbott Laboratories. This checklist was developed as a brief risk-appraisal questionnaire to identify conditions that have the potential to place an individual at nutritional risk (Barrocas, White, Gomez, & Smithwick, 1996). Scores on the ten-item questionnaire range from 0 to 21, with scores of 0 to 2 indicating a good nutritional score; 3 to 5 moderate nutritional risk; and 6 or more high nutritional risk. Posner, Jette, Smith, and Miller (1993) suggest a cut-off of 6 to balance sensitivity and specificity and to reduce the occurrence of misclassifying individuals. Sensitivity is the probability that a person with the disease will have an abnormal (positive) test, whereas specificity is the probability that a person who actually has the disease will have a normal (negative) test result. Posner and colleagues (1993) found that sensitivity was 36%, specificity was 85% and positive predictive value was 38% for a cut-off of 6 points for nutritional risk.

Body Mass Index (BMI)

BMI is defined as body weight in kilograms (kg) divided by the square of height in meters (m), i.e., kg/m^2. For the older adult (age 65 or older), desirable BMI ranges are from 22–27. Indices < 22 are a sign of poor nutrition, and an index > 27 is a major risk factor for obesity (Nutrition Screening Initiative, 1992).

Body Composition (Percentage of Body Fat)

Percentage of body fat was calculated using the TBF 621 Tanita Body Fat Monitor Scales, which is a consumer model. The scale uses Bioelectrical Impedance Analysis (BIA) to screen body fat. The BIA measures resistance to a signal as it travels through the water that is found in fat and muscle. Healthy body fat range, as identified by Tanita, is 17%–23% for males and 20%–27% for females. The consumer model scale has been validated against Dual Energy X-ray Absorptionmetry (DEXA) method (p < 0.001) (Rubiano, Nunez, & Heymsfield, 1999). The DEXA method is considered the "gold standard" in body composition analysis (Tanita Corporation of America, 2000). Individuals with cardiac pacemakers and life supports were excluded from the body fat composition measurement.

Depressive symptoms were assessed using the Center for Epidemiological Studies Depression Scale (CES-D), developed by the National Institute of Mental Health Center for use in general population surveys (Radloff, 1977). The scale is designed to measure current level of depressive symptoms, with emphasis on depressive mood (Himmelfarb & Murrell, 1983; Radloff, 1977).

The Likert-type scale has 20 items related to the frequency of depression over the last week. A 4-point response format is used. Scores range from 0 to 60, with high scores indicating depression. Himmelfarb and Murrell (1983) suggest that an appropriate cut-off for older adults is 20. Penninx, Leveille, Ferrucci, van Eijk, and Guralnik (1999) suggest that a cut-off of 20 offers a more stringent approach to the classification of depressed mood for the older adult. Radloff (1977) found a correlation of 0.56 with a clinical rating of severity of depression and alpha coefficients of .85 for general population samples and .90 for a patient sample. Split-half reliability ranged from 0.76 to 0.85.

The level of physical performance was measured by an 8-foot timed walk score. The timed-walk measures the number of seconds required to ambulate a distance of 8 feet at usual speed while using assistive devices (Martin, 1996). Guralnik, Branch, Cummings, and Curb (1989) suggest that performance tests that are timed, such as walking eight feet or opening a fastener, may be more reproducible and able to measure small changes than self-report or categorical measurements.

Participants were given two opportunities to walk a distance of eight feet, indicated by taped marks on the floor. Participants were instructed to walk at their usual or regular pace, as if they were walking down the hall to their mailbox. Participants used assistive devices such as canes or walkers if needed. Lower scores reflect higher levels of physical performance (Martin, 1996; Seeman et al., 1994).

DESCRIPTION OF INTERVENTIONS

Nutrition education and exercise were the two interventions that were evaluated. All residents of the housing complex had the opportunity to participate in both interventions.

Nutrition educational sessions were held to provide information about factors that increase nutritional risk and to encourage healthy dietary choices. These sessions were conducted by a nutritionist from the local agricultural extension office at the apartment complex every two-weeks for one-hour periods, for a total of four sessions during the eight-week intervention period. Sessions were listed on the monthly activity calendar for the residents and scheduled at 10:00 a.m. or 2:00 p.m. Topics included "The Food Pyramid," "Making Healthy Food Choices on a Limited Budget," "Food Safety Tips," and "Sodium and Where You Find It." Door prizes and refreshments were provided at each session. Average attendance at each session included 13 individuals. Time of day did not affect attendance; however, sending reminders a day before each session stimulated attendance.

Exercise and movement interventions consisted of two types of activities that employed the use of large muscle groups. The purpose of these interventions was to enhance endurance and strength needed to maintain independence. Participants were asked to exercise for 30 minutes three times a week during the eight-week intervention period. Prior to participation in the exercise component, each participant signed a release form. In addition, a registered nurse provided exercise and safety information to the residents before the exercise program was initiated. Participants were instructed to adjust their activity based on pain, fatigue, or physical discomfort.

Exercise and movement activities included chair exercises and walking. Chair exercises consisted of stretching, coordinated movement, and strength building exercises for 20 minutes per session using the video, *Armchair Fitness: Strength Improvement* (CC-M Productions). Each 20-minute session took place on alternate days and included five minutes of warm-up and cool-down activities. Members of the exercise group assisted in preparing the room, setting up the video, and leading the sessions.

Participants were encouraged to walk for 30 minutes at their own speed three days a week and to use assistive devices if needed. Participants walked laps inside the building, outside the apartment building, or at a local park. If necessary, these walking sessions could be divided, leading to an accumulation of 30 minutes of walking per day (Burns, 1996; USDHHS, 2000).

RECRUITMENT PROTOCOL

Following IRB approval, a flyer announcing a meeting to discuss the research project was posted at the site. The meeting was conducted in the community room of the facility by the principal investigator. Refreshments were provided for the meeting and all residents were invited to attend the meeting to consider participation in the study. Data collection began after informed consent was obtained.

DATA COLLECTION

Face-to-face interviews were conducted in the community room of the facility or in the participant's apartment. Interview assessments were conducted in the following order: demographic sheet, nutrition checklist, CES-D, and timed walk. Weight and percentage of body fat measurements were taken for all on two pre-announced days from four to five o'clock in the investigator's office. Individuals with cardiac pacemakers and life ports ($n = 3$) were excluded from the body fat measurement. Weight was obtained using a Healthometer scale. The data collection process required an average of 15 to 20 minutes for each participant.

DATA ANALYSIS

Pretest and post-test data were transferred from the instruments to a Microsoft Excel spreadsheet. The Statview statistical package was used to compute analyses. Unless otherwise stated, a liberal *a priori* level of statistical significance of $p < .10$ was set. To reduce the likelihood of committing a Type II error and to detect trends, a significance level of .10 was chosen.

Descriptive statistics were used to describe the sample prior to initiating interventions. Analyses of variance (ANOVA) and Fisher's PLSD tests were used to compare nutrition scores by levels of participation in the nutrition education intervention. ANOVA and Mann-Whitney Rank tests were used to compare timed-walk scores and depression score change by level of participation in chair exercise, walking exercise, and combined chair and walking exercise group.

RESULTS

Demographic characteristics of the participants are displayed in Table 12.1. Further analysis of the DETERMINE checklist scores indicated that for the sample ($N = 27$), 26% ($n = 7$) had a score between 0 and 2; 52% ($n = 14$) had a score between 3 and 5; and 22% ($n = 6$) had a score ≥ 6. Eighty-nine percent ($n = 24$) of the participants had a CES-D score ≤ 20.

Analysis of Variance at pretest comparing physical performance and depression scores by level of exercise participation indicated a significant difference between groups at the 95% level ($p < .05$)

TABLE 12.1 Description of Variables (N = 27)

Variable	M + SD	Range
BMI	28.70 ± 5.59	17.1–38.5
Body Fat (%)	31.50 ± 11.10	9.0–45.0
Timed Walk (sec)	4.07 ± 2.12	1.5–11.4
DETERMINE Score	4.04 ± 2.56	1.0–12.0
CES-D	8.30 ± 2.56	0–40

in walking speed. That is to say, "exercisers" walked faster than "nonexercisers." Findings also indicated a tendency toward significance for differences ($p = .054$) in depression scores between groups with exercisers tending to have lower depression scores. In other words, individuals who exercised reported fewer depressive symptoms.

Correlational analyses were used to examine associations among study variables. The strongest correlation was noted between BMI and percentage of body fat ($r = .82$). Significant correlations were also noted between nutrition scores and CES-D ($r = .76$), 8-foot timed walk and CES-D ($r = .56$) and 8-foot timed walk and nutrition ($r = .42$).

Nutritional Risk

Descriptive analyses for the sample ($n = 24$) indicate a reduction in the nutrition score mean from pretest to posttest (pretest score $M = 4.04$; posttest score $M = 3.17$). Distribution of post-test scores on the checklist for the sample ($n = 24$) was 38% ($n = 9$) had scores between 0 and 2; 46% ($n = 11$) had scores between 3 and 5; and 17% ($n = 4$) had scores ≥ 6. A reduction in weight also occurred, as did BMI. However, the percentage of body fat ($n = 20$) increased from 31.5% to 33.2% over the eight-week intervention.

The number of nutritional education sessions attended determined the level of participation and ranged from no meetings (0) to all meetings (4). The ANOVA statistical estimates indicated no significant difference in nutritional risk scores by level of participation ($p = .57$) in the nutrition program. There was, however, a tendency toward significance (p = .11) when comparing participants who attended "0" compared with "2" nutritional education sessions.

Physical Performance Status

Change in timed walk scores by exercise types is shown in Table 12.2. At the completion of the intervention period 83% (n = 20) were participating in an exercise intervention compared with 56% (n = 15) at pretest. Walking was the most popular form of exercise activity reported (n = 18).

Depression

Change in depression scores by exercise types is displayed in Table 12.3. There was a statistically significant difference (p = .07) in depression score change by exercise participation group with the exercise group having lower depression scores. Descriptive analyses indicated a general increase in mean scores on the CES-D scale over the eight-week intervention period. Scores at pretest were 8.30 compared with 10.88 at post-test. Although scores increased, 79% (n = 19) had posttest scores < 20.

ADDITIONAL FINDINGS

Participants' comments suggest that they received benefits from participating in the study such as sleeping better, reducing the use

TABLE 12.2   Change in Timed-Walk Scores by Exercise Type (N = 24)

Group	Pretest M + SD	Post-test M + SD	Score Change (p)
Chair (n = 13)	3.61 ± 0.79	3.89 ± 1.13	.26
No Chair (n = 11)	3.83 ± 2.12	3.76 ± 1.77	–
Walk (n = 18)	3.74 ± 1.65	3.88 ± 1.59	.80
No Walk (n = 6)	3.62 ± 1.14	3.67 ± 0.84	–
Combination (n = 10)	3.58 ± 0.89	3.91 ± 1.29	.24
No Comb. (n = 14)	3.80 ± 1.86	3.77 ± 1.56	–
Exercise Post (n = 20)	3.72 ± 1.56	3.85 ± 1.51	.81
No Exercise Post (n = 4)	3.69 ± 1.46	3.72 ± 1.08	–

TABLE 12.3   Change in Depression Scores by Exercise Type (N = 24)

Group	Pretest M ± SD	Post-test M ± SD	Score Change (p)
Chair (n = 13)	8.39 ± 11.18	12.39 ± 12.93	.82
No Chair (n = 11)	6.22 ± 9.23	9.09 ± 9.54	–
Walk (n = 18)	8.47 ± 11.43	10.67 ± 11.50	.41
No Walk (n = 6)	4.17 ± 3.87	11.50 ± 12.08	–
Combination (n = 10)	9.00 ± 12.65	15.00 ± 13.70	.43
No Comb. (n = 14)	6.24 ± 8.30	7.93 ± 8.78	–
Exercise Post (n = 20)	8.52 ± 10.82	9.85 ± 11.20	.07
No Exercise Post (n = 4)	1.75 ± 0.96	16.00 ± 12.57	–

of laxatives, and walking for longer periods of time when shopping with their families. Others commented that the group support made the exercise worthwhile.

LIMITATIONS

Limitations include small sample size and lack of a control group. The inclusiveness of the program prevented the investigator from establishing a control group. The eight-week intervention period may not have provided a sufficient time period to measure changes in physical function status.

Another limitation was the timing of the nutritional assessment in relation to other nutrition education activities. The nutrition meetings began five months before pretest assessment. Topics covered during the five-month period included "Low-Fat Foods," "Calcium, Why We Need It," "Reading Food Labels," and "Foods with Protein." Participants may have modified nutritional habits prior to the beginning of the study. Therefore, nutritional risk scores might have been higher if measured five months earlier.

The CES-D scores at post-test may have been affected by the World Trade Center attacks which occurred two weeks before the post-test measures were taken. At that time, discussion of war was ubiquitous and the residents were somber, expressing difficulty concentrating on tasks and concern for family, friends, and the country. As participants were completing the CES-D, they shared comments such as "Two weeks ago, I was OK. Now I'm scared. I've cancelled my travel plans. I am very depressed over these attacks" or "Oh, I don't know, I get sad when I think about the attacks at the World Trade Center." Most participants mentioned the World Trade Center attacks or threats of war or biological war when completing the depression scale.

DISCUSSION

This study found 26% of the sample ($N = 27$) at pretest and 38% of the sample ($n = 24$) at post-test had low nutritional risk (scores between 0 and 2) on the DETERMINE checklist. Overall, this sample is at higher nutritional risk than other studies that found approximately 50% of a study population at low nutritional risk (Brunt, Schafer, & Oakland, 1999; Phillips & Read, 1997).

There was a tendency toward improved nutritional risk status for individuals who attended two sessions compared with those who attended none. The two sessions were "Sodium and Where You Find It" and "The Food Pyramid." Sahyoun, Jacques, Dallal, and Russell (1997) suggest focusing nutrition education and dietary modifications on the special needs of older adults. These two topics related to specific needs of the older adult, whereas the other two sessions, "Food Safety Tips" and "Planning a Menu on a Limited Budget," provided general information.

EXERCISE

Results revealed a difference in timed-walk scores at baseline with exercisers walking faster than nonexercisers; however, the specific types of exercise did not effect significant improvement in timed-walk scores. Factors such as exercise behavior and the intensity and duration of the exercise intervention may have influenced the lack of improvement. For instance, an exercise class initiated by a group of residents began six weeks prior to this project. Consequently, some improvement may have occurred prior to the baseline assessment and may be a factor influencing the lack of improvement.

The exercise interventions during this eight-week study were of low to moderate intensity for 30-minute sessions. Other studies utilizing exercise interventions have used higher intensity exercise such as weight training programs and longer exercise periods (Fiatarone et al., 1990; Wallace et al., 1998). Sessions that are 30 minutes in length and at a low to moderate level of intensity may require longer than eight weeks to demonstrate an improvement in physical performance status.

In general, the mean score for the CES-D scale was higher at post-test than pretest, indicating an increase in depressive symptoms. There was no difference in the depression scores in the specific exercise group. Yet, there was a statistically significant difference in depression scores change for individuals that exercised versus those who did not.

IMPLICATIONS FOR PRACTICE

Older rural women are willing to participate in wellness programs and modify behavior to improve health and well-being. Structured exercise programs for older adults should be implemented in diverse settings. Nutrition education should include topics that address the special nutritional needs of older rural women because they are interested in obtaining pertinent information.

RECOMMENDATION FOR FUTURE STUDY

Future studies should include a larger sample size as well as a control group. Further studies should evaluate the effectiveness of the interventions as a home-based program for rural women (Gamm, Hutchison, Dabney, & Dorsey, 2003). In addition, further studies should examine the effectiveness of an interdisciplinary approach to providing health education to women in rural communities. Cost-benefit and efficacy of wellness programs for older rural women must also be analyzed. There is also a need to determine if health promotion programs improve access to health care for women. Finally, it is essential that future studies explore the needs of rural older women such as transportation, education about risk behaviors, and innovative approaches to providing health information and planning health interventions (Gamm, Hutchison, Dabney, & Dorsey, 2003). Findings from such studies are vital to the development of quality, cost effective, efficient services for rural older women.

REFERENCES

Administration on Aging (2001). *Profile of older Americans: 2001.* Retrieved September 9, 2004, from http://research.aarp.org/general/profile_2001.pdf

Agency for Health Care Policy and Research (1996). *Improving health care for rural populations.* Retrieved August 19, 2003, from http://www.ahrq.gov/research/rural.htm

Barrocas, A., White, J. V., Gomez, C., & Smithwick, L. (1996). Assessing health status in the elderly: The Nutrition Screening Initiative. *Journal of Health Care for the Poor and Underserved, 7*(3), 210–218.

Berkman, L. F., Seeman, T. E., Albert, M., Blazer, D., Kahn, R., Mohs, R., et al. (1993). High, usual and impaired functioning in community-dwelling older men and women: Findings from the MacArthur Foundation Research Network on Successful Aging. *Journal of Clinical Epidemiology, 46*(10), 1129–1140.

Bruce, M. L., Seeman, T. E., Merrill, S. S., & Blazer, D. G. (1994). The impact of depressive symptomatology on physical disability: MacArthur studies of successful aging. *American Journal of Public Health, 84*(11), 1796–1799.

Brunt, A. R., Schafer, E., & Oakland, M. J. (1999). The ability of the DETERMINE checklist to predict dietary intake of white, rural, elderly community-dwelling women. *Journal of Nutrition for the Elderly, 18*(3), 1–19.

Burns, K. J. (1996). A new recommendation for physical activity as a means of health promotion. *The Nurse Practitioner, 21*(9), 18–22.

Butler, R. N. (1995). Revolution in longevity. In K. Dychtwald (Ed.), *Healthy aging: Challenges and solutions.* Gaithersburg, MD: Aspen Publishers.

Cassel, C. K. (2001). Successful aging: How increased life expectancy and medical advances are changing geriatric care. *Geriatrics, 56*(1), 35–39.

Eberhardt, M. S., Ingram, D. D., Makuc, D. M., Pamuk, E. R., Freid, V. M., Harper, S. B., et al. (2001). *Urban and rural health chartbook: Health, United States.* Hyattsville, MD: National Center for Health Statistics.

Fiatarone, A., Marks, E. C., Ryan, N. D., Meredith, C. N., Litsitz, L. A., & Evans, W. J. (1990). High-intensity strength training in nonagenarians: Effects on skeletal muscle. *Journal of the American Medical Association, 263*(22), 3029–3034.

Gamm, L. D., Hutchison, L. L, Dabney, B. J., & Dorsey, A. M. (Eds.) (2003). *Rural Healthy People 2010: A companion document to Healthy People 2010.* College Station, TX: The Texas A&M University System Health Science Center.

Guralnik, J. M., Branch, L. G., Cummings, S. R., & Curb, J. D. (1989). Physical performance measures in aging research. *Journal of Gerontology, 44*(5), M141–M146.

Himmelfarb, S., & Murrell, S. A. (1983). Reliability and validity of five mental health scales in older persons. *Journal of Gerontology, 38*(3), 333–339.

Johnson, J. E. (1991). Health-care practices of the rural aged. *Journal of Gerontological Nursing, 17*(8), 15–19.

King, A. C., Pruitt, L. A., Phillips, W., Oka, R., Rodenburg, A., & Haskell, W. L. (2000). Comparative effects of two physical activity programs on measured and perceived physical functioning and other health-related quality of life outcomes in older adults. *The Journal of Gerontology, 55*(2), M74–M83.

Koch, R. W. (2001). The Wellness in Senior Housing (WISH) Project: Its impact on perceived health status of older adults residing in a government subsidized housing community. Unpublished doctoral dissertation. Louisiana State University, New Orleans.

List, M. A., Maskay, M. H., Blumberg, K. G., & Banik, D. M. (1999). You're never too old: A cancer education and risk reduction program for the elderly. *Journal of Cancer Education, 14*(2), 104–108.

Mainous, A. G., & Kohrs, F. P. (1995). A comparison of health status between rural and urban adults. *Journal of Community Health, 20*(5), 423–432.

Martin, J. C. (1996). Determinants of functional health of low-income black women with osteoarthritis. *American Journal of Preventive Medicine, 12*(5), 430–436.

McCarron, D. A., Oparil, S., Chait, A., Haynes, B., Kris-Etherton, P., Stern, J. S., et al. (1997). Nutritional management of cardiovascular risk factors: A randomized clinical trial. *Archives of Internal Medicine, 157*(2), 169–177.

Nutrition Screening Initiative (1992). *Nutrition Interventions Manual for Professionals Caring for Older Americans.* Washington, DC: Author.

Ormond, B. A., Wallin, S., & Goldenson, S. M. (2000). *Supporting the rural health care safety net.* Washington, DC: The Urban Institute.

Penninx, B. W. J., Leveille, S., Ferrucci, L., van Eijk, J. T. M., & Guralnik, J. (1999). Exploring the effect of depression on physical disability: Longitudinal evidence from the established populations for epidemiologic studies of the elderly. *American Journal of Public Health, 89*(9), 1346–1352.

Phillips, B. E., & Read, M. H. (1997). Malnutrition in the elderly: A comparison of two nutrition screening methods. *Journal of Nutrition for the Elderly, 17*(1), 39–48.

Posner, B. M., Jette, A. M., Smith, K. W., & Miller, D. R. (1993). Nutrition and health risks in the elderly: The Nutrition Screening Initiative. *American Journal of Public Health, 83*(7), 972–978.

Radloff, L. S. (1977). The CES-D scale: A self-report depression scale for research in the general population. *Applied Psychological Measurement, 1*(3), 385–401.

Rosenthal, T. C., & Fox, C. (2000). Access to health care for the rural elderly. *Journal of the American Medical Association, 284*(16), 2034–2036.

Rowe, J. W., & Kahn, R. L. (1997). Successful aging. *Gerontologist, 37*(4), 433–440.

Rowe, J. W., & Kahn, R. L. (1998). *Successful aging.* New York: Dell Publishing.

Rubiano, F., Nunez, C., & Heymsfield, S. B. (1999). Validity of consumer model bioimpedance analysis system with established dual energy x-ray absoptiometry (DXA). *Medicine and Science in Sports Exercise, 31*(5), 202.

Sahyoun, R., Jacques, P. F., Dallal, G. E., & Russell, R. M. (1997). Nutrition screening initiative checklist may be better awareness/educational tool than screening one. *Journal of the American Dietetic Association, 97*(7), 760–764.

Saunders, C. S. (1999). Hale, not frail: Successful aging. *Patient Care, 33*(8), 162–191.

Seeman, T. E., Berkman, L. F., Charpentier, P. A., Blazer, D. G., Albert, M. S., & Tinetti, M. E. (1995). Behavioral and psychosocial predictors of physical performance: MacArthur studies of successful aging. *Journal of Gerontology: Medical Science, 50A*(4), M177–M183.

Seeman, T. E., Charpentier, P. A., Berkman, L. F., Tinetti, M. E., Guralnik, J. M., Albert, M., et al. (1994). Predicting changes in physical performance in a high-functioning elderly cohort: MacArthur studies of successful aging. *Journal of Gerontology: Medical Science, 49*(3), M97–M108.

Shellman, J. (2000). Promoting elder wellness through a community-based blood pressure clinic. *Public Health Nursing, 17*(4), 257–263.

Tanita Corporation of America (2000). *Understanding body fat analysis.*: Arlington Heights, IL: Author.

Teri, L., McCurry, S. M., & Logsdon, R. G. (1997). Memory, thinking, and aging: What we know about what we know. *Western Journal of Medicine, 167*(4), 269–275.

U.S. Congress, Office of Technology Assessment (1990, September). *Health care in rural America* (OTA-H-434). Washington, DC: U.S. Government Printing Office.

U.S. Department of Health and Human Services (2000). *Healthy People 2010: Understanding and improving health* (2nd ed.). Washington, DC: U.S. Government Printing Office.

Wallace, J. I., Buchner, D. M., Grothaus, L., Leveille, S., Tyll, L., LaCroix, A. Z., et al. (1998). Implementation and effectiveness of a community-based health promotion program for older adults. *The Journal of Gerontology, 53*(4), M301–M306.

Chapter 13

Providing Education and Health Care to Rural Communities Using Telehealth

Denise L. Jameson

BARRIERS TO RURAL HEALTH CARE

Rural health care has unique issues that make the delivery of care problematic. Three fundamental barriers are associated with access to rural health care: critical lack of physicians and other providers, geographic isolation, and hospital solvency.

The rural health system depends on a declining number of hospitals that, when coupled with health professional disincentives to work in rural areas and extensive geographic isolation, creates considerable barriers for rural residents to receive adequate health care services. As a result of these barriers, 75 percent of rural counties in the United States are designated as Medically Underserved Areas (MUA), a measure that includes both provider shortages and poorer health outcomes (Arizona Health Care Cost Containment System, 2001).

Access to quality health care strengthens rural communities. Health care is oftentimes the largest employer in a community, which

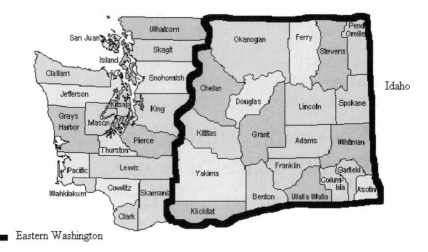

■ Eastern Washington

FIGURE 13.1   Our service area—eastern Washington.

not only impacts the quality of health care but also the financial health of that community. Collaboration is the key to survival in rural communities across America.

OUR SERVICE AREA

Spokane is the second largest city in the state of Washington and home to the second largest hospital in the state and the medical hub of the Inland Northwest, which comprises eastern Washington, northern Idaho, western Montana, and northeast Oregon. The next major medical hub to the east is the Mayo Clinic in Minnesota, 1,380 miles away.

The climate of eastern Washington is varied. In the summer, temperatures can average 95° in the desert areas, whereas it may drop to freezing in the high wilderness mountains, creating a haven for summer boaters, campers, hikers, and fishermen. This infusion of summer vacationers brings thousands of dollars into the community along with added stress on the small medical community.

The winter months are different. Several mountain passes in the region, including one that links eastern and western Washington are subject to frequent closures due to snow. This heavy snowfall brings winter sports to the region, but also isolates some communities from access to food, shelter, and healthcare.

According to the Health Policy Administration Program (2002) " . . . one of every four residents lives in a rural community, and their access to health care is, as a result, at risk. Consider these indicators:

- Residents in rural eastern Washington are 1.4 times more likely to be uninsured than the state's average, 13.4% versus 9.5%. Moreover, 14.7% of children in those rural areas have no insurance, nearly double the statewide average.

- Rural residents have lower incomes, are older, and have less education on average, all of which are related to higher levels of illness and injury and, thus, demands on providers.

- Employment-based insurance is less prevalent in rural Washington, because higher percentages of people in those communities are self-employed, work for small businesses, or do seasonal work."

Fig. 13.1 shows out service area in rural eastern Washington which covers 60% of the state's total landmass. The state is 66,581 square miles and eastern Washington is 38,946 square miles, yet it houses only 18.5% of the total state population. Eastern Washington includes nineteen counties with a total population of 669,848, including Spokane County with a population of 417,939. Children age 0 to 18 comprise about 28% of the population, compared with 26% statewide, and seniors age 65 and over comprise 13.5% of the population, compared with less than 12% statewide (Access Washington, 2004). Since eastern Washington is predominantly agricultural in nature, the area has a large population of migrant farm workers that transition in and out of the communities with seasonal employment opportunities.

As emphasized by *Healthy People 2010*, economic status plays a role in adequate nutrition, housing, and health care purchasing power, all of which affect the quality of health. In addition, there is a close correlation between poverty and unhealthy behaviors and disease (U.S. Department of Health and Human Services, 2000). The economic prosperity that Washington's urban areas have enjoyed in recent years has left its rural areas far behind, as the State has one of the largest economic gaps between urban and rural areas in the nation. Incomes in most of the rural counties in eastern Washington rank solidly in the bottom half among all counties in the State, some at least 10% below the state average. The state of the economy is even grimmer when considering the percentage of the population enrolled in Medicaid. Currently 35% of the population in Adams County is on medical assistance, the highest percentage of any county in the State (Office of Financial Management, n.d.).

SOLUTION

In order to fulfill the growing health care needs of this 39,946 square mile area, Inland Northwest Health Services (INHS), has become the largest health care delivery system in the nation that meets both rural and urban areas, outside the Veterans Administration. Five Spokane hospitals—Deaconess Medical Center, Holy Family Hospital, Sacred Heart Medical Center, St. Luke's Rehabilitation Institute, Valley Hospital and Medical Center; Mount Carmel Hospital in Colville and Kootenai Medical Center in Coeur d'Alene, Idaho—were distinguished as being among the most technologically superior health care institutions in the nation. *Hospital and Health Networks*, the journal of the American Hospital Association, surveyed more than 1,100 hospitals to name the *100 Most Wired* hospitals and health systems in the *2003 Most Wired Survey and Benchmarking Study*. As Fred Galusha, Chief Information Officer at INHS has stated, "We are continuing to reaffirm the important role collaboration plays in the delivery of health care information through the development of new technologies. We are pleased the rest of the country is taking notice of our innovation in the Inland Northwest."

How does being "wired" connect rural communities with services available at urban sites? It provides education and access to medical specialists through state-of-the-art technology and links urban and rural facilities through various mediums and services.

INHS provides education for the community and health care workers in the following areas: prenatal classes, diabetes education, and pediatric trauma; clinical consults on such specialties as dermatology, radiology, and nephrology; physician continuing education classes; and hospital and prehospital courses on natural disasters, mass casualty incidents, communicable diseases, and bioterrorist events.

THE CREATION OF INLAND NORTHWEST HEALTH SERVICES

Hindsight is defined as the "perception of the significance and nature of events after they have occurred." That is what we now know about the creation of INHS. For example, a review of urban hospitals that closed between 1990 and 2000 revealed that nationally:

- Generally, urban hospital closures resulted from competition, business-related decisions, or a low number of patients.

- Hospital services were still available within 10 miles from most of the urban hospitals that closed (Department of Social and Health Services, 2003).

Year 2000 data obtained from the Washington State Department of Health show the average hospital-operating margin to be barely above zero. This margin is far below the four to five percent needed for financial health (Yellowlees, 2000).

> The rise of consumerism with more importance being placed on patients that are informed about their disorders, means that there will have to be more collaboration with patients in the future and greater focus within health care systems on providing distributed care, better access, choice, and equity for patients, in a distributed manner close to their homes (Hasnain-Wynia, Margolin, & Bazzoli, 2001).

Thus, collaborative efforts are considered a powerful means of improving community health.

We now know that for the above foresight in 1994, Spokane hospitals needed to change things which prompted the formation of INHS, a 501(c)(3) nonprofit corporation. Both hospital systems owned an air medical transport system, provided community education, and individually maintained a computer network including medical records, billing, etc. Each hospital also provided medical transportation of clients and there was no referral system available for rural physicians. All of these services were costing the hospitals millions in lost revenue.

INHS began in 1994 as a collaborative effort between Empire Health Services and Providence Services of Eastern Washington (sponsoring entities), the management companies of Deaconess and

Valley Hospitals, and Sacred Heart and Holy Family Hospitals. These companies were, and still are, major competitors, but they put the competition aside to create INHS in order to more efficiently provide better patient care at a better price for the entire four-state Inland Northwest region. INHS didn't happen overnight. After years of care from its Board of Directors, the first management team came on board in 1998. INHS personnel and programs were scattered through the various hospitals and other leased space until their move into the historic Holley Mason Building in October 2001. INHS occupies two entire floors at the Holley Mason, and their facility includes a state-of-the-art information resource management center with a 24/7 help desk that served 30,000 clients in 2002.

The two organizations with individual philosophies joined together to reduce duplication and improve quality of services to the community. Kramer (1991) states that for any merger or affiliation to be a success, it must produce market and financial advantages for the new partnerships and offer the community a significant improvement in quality of care and services. Furthermore, partnerships can enhance organizational and personal relationships in the community and thus promote the health of residents (Hasnain-Wynia, Margolin, & Bazzoli, 2001).

The INHS structure is an example of a centralized action model. In this structure the partnership is a formal and a self-contained entity, with a dedicated staff that are paid through partnership funds (Hasnain-Wynia, Margolin, & Bazzoli, 2001). INHS currently employs 850 individuals who coordinate a variety of services to hospitals representing 2,880 beds. The executive director manages INHS and reports to a board of directors comprising eight members of the sponsoring entities' group boards, respective CEOs, and other medical and community professionals. INHS oversees a variety of health care divisions and services. Partnership funding supports some of the services and others are self-supporting or grant funded. These services are described in Table 13.1.

The persistence and vision of the sponsoring health care organizations has created a state of the art health care system for the residents of eastern Washington and a model for the nation. What does this mean? How does it work? Here is an example of what any person living or visiting our state can expect:

> Imagine Angela going on a much needed retreat to the far reaches
> of Washington State and suffering an unexpected accident in a

TABLE 13.1   Divisions of Inland Northwest Health Services

Service	Activity
Children's Miracle Network (CMN)	• Raises awareness and funds for pediatric services • Includes 10 urban and rural hospitals
Community Health Education and Resources (CHER)	• Provides public and professional educational courses at urban hospitals and to rural hospitals over telehealth
Information Resource Management (IRM)	• System security, medical modules, web systems, internet/intranet, and e-mail to 33 hospitals • Over 2,000,000 medical records on network available to 33 hospitals
Northwest MedStar	• Critical care air ambulance service • Service area includes Washington, Oregon, Idaho, Montana, and some flights to Canada and the eastern U.S. • Provides trauma education to all first responders and medical personnel in service area • 3,000 patients transported in 2002
Northwest MedVan	• Medical transport service for those that do not have transportation to medical appointments • 21,000 individuals served in 2002
Northwest TeleHealth	• Videoconferencing for 42 hospitals and/or mental health centers, clinics, and correctional facilities in both urban and rural settings • Includes clinical consultations, federal and state satellite broadcasts, community and medical personnel education offerings, statewide meetings and trainings
Spokane Med Direct	• Toll-free medical referral system • Links rural medical providers with urban specialists • 7,000 calls in 2002
St. Luke's Rehabilitation Institute	• Largest freestanding medical rehabilitation center in Washington, northern Idaho, and Montana

rural area at night. She is taken to a local hospital, which has limited trauma response capabilities and has to be transported to Spokane. Time is of the essence and there are no surgeons, anesthesiologists, pharmacists or specialists at the local hospital. This situation is commonplace in many rural areas of Washington and is compounded by the necessity of traveling great distances to reach specialized care. Following recent events, Washington state and the rest of the country have come to understand the need to be more prepared for potential emergencies, natural disasters and to have in place the necessary alert mechanisms.

Now, how do all of INHS's services assist in this situation?

MedStar is dispatched to the town of Republic, a 50-minute flight. While getting the plane ready, trauma specialists, over TeleHealth, review her medical records from visits to an urban hospital in the past and current medical and laboratory records at the rural hospital, along with educational classes attended through CHER, then direct clinicians on the safe "packaging" of a patient for transport. While the patient is waiting for MedStar, medical personnel in Republic are teleconferencing with a neurologist in Spokane using TeleHealth concerning the specialized care needed to ensure that the patient is receiving all of the necessary lifesaving care without delays. While vital signs are monitored, blood drawn, and x-rays taken, information is entered into a shared medical records system where the neurologists are reading the results as they are entered. The patient arrives in Spokane and the continuum of care remains unbroken.

Below is a description of two of the INHS collaborative efforts that serve rural communities and their health care facilities.

Northwest TeleHealth

Telemedicine is a technological fix for the uneven distribution or inefficient allocation of health care services, both geographically and temporally (Grigsby, 2002). Telehealth uses communications and computer technologies to transfer medical information and expertise for clinical, educational, research, and administrative applications. The terms *telehealth* and *telemedicine* are often used interchangeably, but telemedicine only refers to the portion of telehealth that is focused on patient care (American Telemedicine Association, 1999).

In 1997, INHS obtained funding through the Office for the Advancement of TeleHealth (OAT) to expand telehealth services. In 2002, network services have expanded to 42 urban and rural hospitals, physician's offices, clinics, Regional Support Networks (RSNs), and prisons, providing clinical consultations, community education, and access to specialists through teleconferencing. This means a patient can see a specialist in another city without leaving his or her community.

The network is also in a pilot project through the Office for the Advancement of TeleHealth which hopes to demonstrate the efficacy of linking an urban trauma center to three rural hospital emergency rooms to provide an additional level of support to providers and patients. The program also has the potential to provide access to other services such as wound care and professional medical education.

Telemedicine capabilities can be as small or large as needed. Five years ago a large telehealth system cost close to $300,000. Today, with improvements in technology, innovations in data compression, and reductions in computing costs, the expense of the equipment required to conduct telemedicine consultations can be less than $5,000 (American Telemedicine Association, 1999). The smaller system can include a simple video camera attached to a physician's computer and linked to a telehealth system at a rural site.

Northwest TeleHealth services have saved Washington rural residents and hospitals hundreds of thousands of dollars. For connected sites, the Northwest Telehealth website (www.nwtelehealth. org) provides online registration, a calendar of events, and reporting on usage, attendance, and cost savings. A calendar of global events and other services are available to the public. For medical personnel using telehealth capabilities, online data tracking tools include the immediate reporting of events entered into the calendar system, and simultaneously calculates cost savings related to unnecessary travel time, mileage reimbursement of personnel, meal expense, lodging due to distance, and, if necessary, replacement personnel.

In 2002, at the request of the Washington State Department of Health, INHS facilitated the preparation of a regional bioterrorism plan for 22 urban and rural hospitals. The use of telehealth enabled these small hospitals to alleviate the necessity to send staff up to 200 miles away to participate in meetings. The tracking tool has estimated cost savings to rural hospitals for these meetings at $83,000.

The American Telemedicine Association reports that the future of telehealth has three focal points:

1.   An Export Service—Residents of many nations have substandard access to specialty health care. Because of the innovations in computing and telecommunications technology,

many elements of health care can be accomplished when the provider and the recipient are geographically separated. This separation could be across town, across a state, or across continents.

To address this focal point, Northwest TeleHealth has migrated to the Western side of Washington to facilitate statewide meetings and provide mental health services between seven out of nine mental health RSNs. Washington's proximity to Canada, Western Montana, and Northern Idaho demonstrates that the possibilities of expanding services into vast rural areas are limitless.

2.   Homecare—Telehomecare has probably one of the greatest potentials for rapid growth worldwide. In the past decade the home monitoring industry has developed electronic and telecommunication equipment which enables medical care to be provided using telemedicine techniques rather than relying on in-person care to patients in their homes.

To address this focal point, Northwest TeleHealth began working with local home health care agencies in 2001 to provide home video monitors for nurses to place in patient's homes. The nurses were able to connect with the clients and provide education and follow-up without leaving the office.

3.   Internet—The next logical step is to deliver health care using the Internet. This is happening in small steps today, but we are poised for it to become a major factor in the delivery of health care over the next five years.

To address this final focal point, INHS' IRM Department employs over 130 technical specialists who have assisted in the implementation of a medical records system and modules that provide linkage with all 33 hospitals. IRM provides ongoing technical assistance to the rural and urban hospitals. There are currently 2,075,000 patients on INHS's secure system.

Spokane is ready to emerge as a major player in providing consultations, diagnoses, treatment, and delivery of prescription medications online. This opens the potential for horizontal monopolies for health care—the virtual online medical system.

"Today, patients accept the use of assessment and treatment on video systems easily" (Yellowlees, 2000). Often in the rural setting, this is the only option for treatment. Clinical services offered over telehealth to the rural communities of eastern Washington and northern Idaho include: Behavioral Health, Cardiology, Case Management/ Discharge Planning, Dermatology, Grand Rounds (Tumor Board, Breast Tumor Board, OB/GYN Board, Genetics, Pediatrics and Psychiatry), Provider Education, Emergency, Neurology, Pediatrics, Psychiatry, Post-Surgical Assessment, Rehabilitation Therapy, and Consultation and Follow-Ups.

Telehealth also offers clinical education programs including Continuing Medical Education programs for physicians, Advanced Cardiac Life Support, Emergency Medical Technician training, and nursing education. TelePharmacy capabilities were recently added to link an urban tertiary hospital with three rural eastern Washington hospitals. This milestone allows patients at a rural hospital pharmacy to receive needed medication through a dispensing machine authorized by a pharmacist in Spokane, 24 hours a day, seven days a week. This service offers a solution to the critical shortage of hospital pharmacists in underserved rural areas of Washington. The program also addresses preventable medication errors that result in an average hospital cost of $4,700 per admission (Kohn, Corrigan, & Donaldson, 1999) and the cost of a pharmacist's salary, if one could be recruited.

Community Health Education and Resources

In 1997 all Spokane hospital educational services were combined into INHS, and CHER was formed by consolidation of Spokane's four hospital community education departments for the purpose of working together to improve the overall health status of the community. This collaboration decreased the redundancies being experienced by the major hospital systems in the community, saved money, and improved access to health care across the community. Programs are rotated from hospital to hospital, thus eliminating "favoritism." Most urban educational classes are available over telehealth.

Educating patients about their diseases and providing health promotion information improves outcomes (Farquhar, Behnke, Detels, & Albright, 1997) and by educating and empowering patients to participate in their own health decisions, the health care system can save money (Behnke, Farquhar, Detels, & Bertram, 1997). Our sponsoring entities have supported and provided health education to the community since their creation, nearly 100 years ago. They realized that if they collaborated, more services would result and the health of the community would continue to improve.

In 2002, CHER served 20,894 local and regional residents. Many of the programs such as public forums and health screenings are free because of funding from the hospitals. Other class expenses are covered through revenue collected from private payors, insurance, and Medicaid/Medicare. Grant opportunities are always being explored to increase funding to provide services.

In eastern Washington, hospitals have provided community education, and they have often been the primary providers of health education to their patients. Through CHER, the Spokane area hospitals offer professional instructors and materials, affordable programs, and a wide variety of preventative education and disease management. The majority of CHER programs are offered in a group setting with opportunities for questions and group discussions. In a study using focus groups of rural women to get input about cardiovascular health, the women reported their preferred learning experiences were those that are hands-on, combined with classes where group members would help motivate and support each other (Krummel, Humphries, & Tessaro, 2002). In a telephone survey of 1,000 HMO clients, over half of the women reported interest in attending group classes of one or more sessions (Thompson & Nussbaum, 2000).

All of CHER's classes and screenings are reviewed for their importance and role in the community's health education continuum. Program goals are identified through feedback received from previous events and classes and through interviews with key health care education leaders. Screenings and classes have an evaluation at the end of each session. The evaluation process includes a questionnaire from attendees and evaluation forms from instructors and speakers involved in the events with the goal of making adjustments for future programs. Input from the evaluations along with the number of participants is used to determine whether or not to continue to offer the program, class, or event. This process gives CHER an opportunity to adjust to changing perceptions about health, learning needs, and the changing mediums necessary to communicate with the target audiences for these programs.

Spanier (2001) has observed that "the rural population makes up about 20% of U.S. citizens, but is served by only about 10% of the nation's physicians." Therefore, universities need to include learners of many different circumstances, to place them at the center of learning communities, and to be committed to meeting their needs, wherever they are. This is also a goal of hospitals and community health education providers, all of whom must continue to explore ways to take urban health education opportunities into our rural communities.

CHER received funds from a Vitamins Antitrust Settlement (Washington State Office of the Attorney General, 2005) to provide education to women with diabetes. The goals were to provide information to health professionals and their clients about the importance of good blood glucose control as well as the need for folic acid supplements. Rural communities, using telehealth, were the targeted population.

CHER was also one of four organizations nationwide to receive a Latino Influencer Network grant to provide diabetes education to clients in the city of Othello, Washington, located 116 miles southwest of Spokane. This city has a population of 16,238. Of this number, 47% are Latino. The primary means of employment are agriculture and shift-work at a major potato processing plant. Residents are served by a community hospital and community clinic. INHS has telehealth equipment at the 49-bed hospital connected to larger urban facilities. Diabetes education along with other specialized medical care is not available to this rural, isolated community.

As a recipient of the Latino Influencer Network grant, a continuing education program was offered to health care providers at no cost. Nine rural sites were connected to the presentation. A perinatologist based in Spokane provided critical education to many rural sites through one presentation. Grant opportunities continue to be explored to provide patients as well as health care providers continuing education in their own communities.

CHER offers community health education through the use of the Telehealth system in an effort to bring health education services to individuals that wouldn't otherwise have access to them. Programs offered over Telehealth include Diabetes Self-Management,

Health and Lifestyle, Babysitting, and Tobacco Cessation. Prepared Childbirth and Basic Life Support are two additional programs CHER will be expanding to offer via Telehealth.

RESEARCH BASED EVIDENCE OF THE BENEFITS OF PROVIDING EDUCATION TO COMMUNITIES USING TELECONFERENCING EQUIPMENT

In many settings the services offered by Northwest TeleHealth and CHER would not be available. This is often true in many rural communities throughout the United States (Yellowlees, 2000). In 2000, an evaluation was done on a telehealth project in Brisbane, Australia, for 13 rural sites in northern Queensland. All the sessions were interactive and viewers were able to address questions to the speakers. Feedback from the evaluation forms showed that over 95% of the participants found the program informative and interesting, and 96% found videoconferencing to be a suitable method for health education and would attend another seminar in the future. The women also reported valuing the opportunity to obtain information within their own communities and not having to travel (Faulkner, 2001).

A five-year collaboration was begun with University of Texas Medical Branch in Galveston School of Nursing and the Lamar University Department of Nursing in Beaumont, Texas. They worked together to establish a telehealth clinic for children with disabling health conditions. They report their observation that one of the primary benefits was that using telecommunications facilitated a multidisciplinary approach to client care. In addition, the long commute and the need to rearrange work schedules had limited the number of family members and/or care providers who could accompany the client to a clinic visit. In the telehealth clinic, it was observed that the client was often accompanied by community health and school nurses, teachers, school principals, or other health care providers. The children were not intimidated by the technology and most were enthralled with being on TV (Green et al., 2000).

Comfort of use by patients and bringing the team together when teleheatlh is used has been shown to be true in CHER's programs. Two certified diabetes educators provided diabetes education to a

5-year-old in a rural setting. The mother, a social worker, a clinic nurse, and an interpreter were all present at the consultation. The child was watching the TV so intently and was not intimidated in the least. The health care team, which included the mother, was able to provide feedback and decide on goals together.

CHALLENGES

The biggest challenge in the creation of INHS was employee retention. Spokane has a high employee retention rate, one reason being there are not a lot of places to "move around" in careers. The first duplicated services to be combined were Heartflight and Lifebird, which became one on August 28, 1994 and are now known as Northwest MedStar. However, no one thought of the details that might be necessary to combine two competing organizations. One detail would be standardization of uniforms. Employees of each organization continued to wear their uniforms from their previous employer. Another detail was location. The combined organizations did not combine their headquarters into one location until 1997. (We are happy to report, however, that the chief flight nurse of Heartflight is now the director of Northwest Medstar.)

There are no challenges in providing educational classes to rural sites over telehealth. The only limitation may be the hands-on classes, i.e., CPR, that are not possible using a teleconferencing medium. For both telehealth and CHER there are no legal challenges. INHS employs a full-time HIPAA Coordinator. All programs and services are approved by the coordinator in advance and all proper compliance documentation is administered.

Nevertheless, there are two major telehealth challenges remaining.

Financial

The cost of the equipment at a site is minimal. Rural sites receive Universal Service Fund reimbursement for a percentage of their monthly T1 line costs. However, this percentage does not cover the entire cost. Bridging the digital divide is still a serious concern for rural America. In many areas the cost of installing a T1 line is expensive or even prohibitive. At times, the financial means of rural hospitals make it impossible for them to continue the use of teleconferencing equipment, which, in turn, impacts the sustainability of continued access to specialized medical services.

Clinical

States have different rules and requirements for the reimbursement of clinical services over telehealth. The largest barrier to the clinical use of telehealth is the lack of reimbursement for certain clinical diagnoses.

Supported by research, Grigsby reports that one barrier to telehealth growth is caused by financial difficulties. There is a lack of reimbursement for specialists, a lack of long-term funding sources, exorbitant telecommunications costs, and lack of or inadequate Medicare reimbursement. Therefore it seems likely that growth will likely follow funding conduits rather than the information superhighway (Grigsby, 2002). INHS is challenged to continue to evaluate funding sources and examine ways for telehealth to be financially sustainable. Discussions must occur with third-party payors to reimburse for telehealth in the same way any other service is reimbursed. The American Telemedicine Association states that the hurdles for telehealth include legal and regulatory barriers and acceptance of the use of telemedicine by traditional medical establishments (American Telemedicine Association, 1999).

CONCLUSION

It is clear that the health care industry is faced with many challenges. Rising costs, increasing demands, and decreasing resources in rural communities provide opportunities for more and better collaboration. The Washington State Hospital Association reports that as hospitals face continuing financial problems, some of the services that benefit the community must be eliminated. Access to health care may, therefore, become threatened in their communities. Inland Northwest Health Services is an example of rising to face that challenge. With the support of hospital systems collaborating instead of competing, the INHS can continue to offer cost-effective, high-quality medical care.

Copeland (1993) believes that the time is ripe for a new philosophy and new opportunities on behalf of health care consumers. "The time is at hand for a new American Revolution; one based on educated health care consumers." The American Telemedicine Association reports that the promise of telemedicine is providing improved and cost effective access to health care and is helping to transform the delivery of health care and improve the health of millions of people throughout the world (American Telemedicine Association, 1999). In this chapter we have shown how Spokane, Washington is an example of an urban city collaborating with health care providers to educate, provide medical care, and use new resources to transform the delivery of health care. Two competing hospital systems have chosen to come together to improve the health care of the community and have more resources to reach the surrounding rural areas.

REFERENCES

Access Washington (n.d.). Retrieved October 8, 2004, from http://access.wa.gov/government/awgeneral.aspx

American Telemedicine Association. "Telemedicine: A Brief Overview" developed for the Congressional Telehealth Briefing, June 23, 1999, Retrieved September 8, 2003 from http://www.atmeda.org/whatis/whitepaper.html

Arizona Health Care Cost Containment System (2001). Initiatives to Improve Access to Rural Health Care Services, A Briefing Paper. Retrieved October 8, 2004, from http://www.ahcccs.state.az.us/Studies/HRSAGrant/RuralPaper.pdf

Behnke, K. S., Farquhar, J. W., Detels, M. P., & Bertram, J. (1997). Private sector-funded community health promotion. *American Journal of Health Promotion, 11*(6), 415–416.

Copeland, J. (1993). Health care needs a proconsumer movement. *Business & Health, 11*(7), 80, 79.

Department of Social and Health Services, Office of Inspector General (2003). Trends in Rural Hospital Closure. Retrieved October 11, 2004, from http://www.oig.hhs.gov/oei/reports/oei-04-02-00610.pdf

Farquhar, J. W., Behnke, K. S., Detels, M. P., & Albright, C. L. (1997). Short and long-term outcomes of a health promotion program in a small rural community. *American Journal of Health Promotion, 11*(6), 411–414.

Faulkner, K. (2001). Successes and failures in videoconferencing: A community health education programme. *Journal of Telemedicine and Telecare, 7*(S2), 65–67.

Green, A., Esperat, C., Seale, D., Chalambaga, M., Smith, S., Walker, et al. (2000). The evolution of a distance education initiative into a major telehealth project. *Nursing and Health Care Perspectives, 21*(2), 66–70.

Grigsby, W. J. (2002). Telehealth: An assessment of growth and distribution, *The Journal of Rural Health, 18*(2), 348–358.

Hasnain-Wynia, R., Margolin, F. S., & Bazzoli, G. J. (2001, May/June). Models for community health partnerships. *Health Forum Journal, 44*(3), 29–33.

Health Policy Administration Program (2000, August). Rural Health Policy: Where do we go from here? Retrieved October 11, 2004, from http://www. users.qwest.net/~wwahec/LandscapeReport.html

Kohn, L., Corrigan, J., & Donaldson, M. (Eds.) (1999). *Why do errors happen? Building a safer health system.* Washington, DC: National Academy Press.

Kramer, R. J. (1991). Partnerships for the future. *Health Progress, 72*(5), 42–45.

Krummel, D. A., Humphries, D., & Tessaro, I. (2002). Focus groups on cardiovascular health in rural women: Implications for practice, *Journal of Nutrition Education and Behavior, 34*(1), 38–46.

Miller, S. L, Reber, R. J., & Chapman-Novakofski, K. (2001). Prevalence of CVD risk factors and impact of a two-year education program for premenopausal women. *Women's Health Issues, 11*(6), 486–493.

Office of Financial Management, State of Washington (n.d.). Population, Economic and Labor Force Information. Retrieved October 8, 2004, from www.ofm.wa.gov

Spanier, G. B. (2001). Bridging rural women's health into the new millennium. *Women's Health Issues, 11*(1), 2–6.

Thompson, M., & Nussbaum, R. (2000). An HMO survey on mass customization of healthcare delivery for women. *Women's Health Issues, 10*(1), 10–11.

U.S. Department of Health and Human Services (2000, November). *Healthy People 2010: Understanding and improving health* (2nd ed.). Washington, DC: U.S. Government Printing Office. Available at http://www.healthypeople.gov/

Washington State Office of the Attorney General. (n.d.). Retrieved April 29, 2005, from http://www.atg.wa.gov/trust/vitamins/cvltr.htm

Yellowlees, P. M. (2000). Telemedicine, e-Health and Global Health Service Delivery in the Third Millennium, Business Briefing Next-Generation Healthcare. Retrieved May 2, 2005 from http://www.wma.net/e/publications/pdf/2000/ yellowlees.pdf

Chapter 14

A Research Agenda for the Future: Linking the Mental, Behavioral, and Physical Health of Rural Women

Luanne E. Thorndyke

The purpose of the conference which formed the basis for this book was to focus attention on rural women's health through the integration of mental, behavioral, and physical components that make up the complex being to which we apply the single identifier "rural woman." It should now be undeniably clear that the term "rural woman" is as complicated as the patchwork quilt that epitomizes her being. Further, it is increasingly obvious that a complete understanding of the health of rural women is not possible without a clear linkage and integration of the biological/psychological/social model of health and disease. Thus, the second national rural women's health conference, specifically identifying the theme "Rural Women's Health: Linking Mental, Behavioral, and Physical Health," has provided significant information to advance our understanding of rural women. What have we learned?

A PATCHWORK OF QUILTED PIECES ON A COMMON BACKGROUND

Women who live in a rural environment are not a homogeneous group. They represent many different ethnic, cultural, and socioeconomic groups. They are of all ages, but increasingly—and disproportionately—old. Although rural women represent approximately 30 percent of the women living in the United States, they are scattered throughout every state in the country.

Despite the diversity of groups who comprise "rural women," the rural environments in which these women live have many characteristics in common, both positive and negative. Mulder and Lambert, in Chapter 1, identify a multitude of challenges that are more significant for rural women as a group than for their urban counterparts. These stressors and challenges fall into three categories: socioeconomic, sociocultural, and physical/emotional. A brief review of each of these areas will provide the framework for understanding the demographics of rural women and rural life.

SOCIOECONOMIC CHALLENGES OF RURAL LIFE

The economic status of rural America is in decline, and rural residents experience the reality of that decline. The rates of poverty are higher and the levels of education are lower than in urban communities. Small rural communities often have limited opportunities for educational advancement or vocational development. Unemployment and a scarcity of economic resources are common in rural communities. These facts highlight the reality of life for rural women as well as rural men.

Women, however, are more severely affected by rural poverty. More than half of rural families with children under 18 years of age have annual incomes below the poverty line (U.S. Department of Agriculture, 2000). Rural families headed by women are nearly four times as likely to be living in poverty and experiencing a greater degree of poverty than are traditional families. Elderly women, often single and/or widowed, are frequently poor. Poverty levels are highest for ethnic minority women, particularly those living in the rural southeastern United States (U.S. Department of Agriculture, 1998).

SOCIOCULTURAL CHALLENGES OF RURAL LIFE

Mulder and Lambert also describe various sociocultural stressors of rural life. These include traditional, patriarchal families with gender-defined work roles and responsibilities, geographic and social isolation, and lack of anonymity. The latter factor may cause a woman experiencing violence in the home or mental health issues to "suffer in silence" rather than seek professional assistance.

The sociocultural role of the rural woman is much more constrained than that of the urban woman. Traditional definitions of wife, mother, and daughter leave little room for women to advance within their communities. In order to partake in educational and vocational opportunities, women (and men) often must leave the community and travel to an urban environment. Those who remain in the rural environment as they progress from childhood to adult life often live in communities with a paucity of economic opportunities. Other community support services, including the health care services of medical primary care providers, specialty services, mental health facilities and workers, and social services are also too often absent in these rural sites.

Counterbalancing these sociocultural factors is the historical legacy left by the frontier settlers of the American west. Self-reliance, independence, heartiness, and rugged resilience characterized the women of these times. These attitudes, with deep historical roots and traditions, have continued to influence rural women. This proud independence can sometimes result in detrimental effects on the health of rural women when it becomes a barrier to seeking needed physical and mental health care services. Rural cultural values, including self-sufficiency and a reluctance to seek medical care unless seriously ill, may influence a rural woman's decision to use health care services.

The paradox of rural life is most apparent in the sociocultural context of communities. Small rural communities are critical to sustaining rural life and to combatting the social isolation of the rural environment. Familiarity, interdependence, shared friendship, and support are positive characteristics of "small town life." However, anonymity is often elusive. As previously stated, the lack of anonymity may have a negative impact on women, who may choose not to seek assistance in situations involving domestic violence, substance abuse, or mental illness.

MEDICAL AND HEALTH CONSIDERATIONS IN RURAL WOMEN

Finally, Mulder and Lambert detail the health differences between rural and urban women. Rural women suffer higher rates of chronic illness and greater morbidity from chronic diseases including diabetes, cancer, hypertension, heart disease, stroke, and lung disease (Centers for Disease Control and Prevention, 1997; Duelberg, 1992; U.S. Department of Agriculture, 1997). Behavioral factors that influence the increased rates of chronic disease include increased rates of smoking and obesity, lack of exercise, and lower rates of preventive care services in rural women compared with urban women. Additional information in particular behavioral areas such as obesity, nutrition, and exercise is detailed in Chapters 4, 9, and 12, and summarized in this chapter. The exception to the general premise that negative behavioral factors lead to increased rates of disease in rural women is discussed in Chapter 9, where Campbell, Bursac, and Perkins found that American Indian Women in Oklahoma, who suffer increased rates of chronic disease and behavioral health risk factors, actually exercise *more* than non-American Indian/Alaska Native women in Oklahoma.

Fetal, infant, and maternal mortality are disproportionately higher in rural areas, as is the rate of teenage pregnancy. The rate of low birthweight is higher among White women living in nonmetropolitan areas (Lishner, Larson, Rosenblatt, & Clark, 1999; Larson, Hart, & Rosenblatt, 1997), though overall crude rates of low birthweight in nonmetropolitan areas are slightly lower than rates in urban areas (Peck & Alexander, 2003). In Chapter 5, Hillemeier, Weisman, Chase, and Romer outline the risk factors for preterm birth and low birthweight among rural women. These include socioeconomic disadvantage, lower educational levels, and an increased risk of exposure to health risks such as smoking, toxic herbicides and pesticides, and higher levels of psychosocial stress. Rural women have reduced access to appropriate medical care, receive fewer screening and preventive services (Casey, Call, & Klingner, 2001), and receive less adequate prenatal care than women in metropolitan environments.

Biobehavioral problems such as domestic violence are as common in rural communities as in urban areas. The occupational hazards of rural employment are unique to the environment and include exposure to agricultural chemicals, with the resultant risk for developing certain cancers and blood disorders. Traumatic injuries from accidents are more common in rural areas, with higher risk of death related to these accidents, due at least in part to lack of accessibility to emergency and trauma care.

ACCESS AND INSURANCE ISSUES

Access to health care services, availability of services (particularly specialty services), and availability and affordability of health insurance are major differentiating features of health care in the rural environment. Mulder and Lambert cite geographic and transportation issues, lack of child care or other coverage, as well as the availability of specialists as barriers. Lack of health insurance and the cost of health care were identified as the most dominant barriers to receiving health care.

The delivery of rural health care is also problematic. There is a critical lack of physicians and other service providers. The rural health system depends on a declining number of hospitals that are threatened by financial insolvency. Geographic isolation, coupled with professional disincentives to work in rural areas, creates significant barriers to rural communities' ability to attract and retain health professionals to serve rural residents.

The disparities between rural and urban areas are most apparent in the arena of access and availability of health care personnel. Physicians and physician specialty services are less available in rural areas, and the distances that must be traveled to obtain these services are greater. Rural communities account for half of the health professional shortage areas (HPSA) in the United States (Health Resources and Services Administration, 2003). Approximately 75 percent of all rural counties in the United States are designated as Medically Underserved Areas (MUAs), a measure that includes both provider shortages and poorer health outcomes (Arizona Health Care Cost Containment System, 2001). Access to mental health service providers such as psychiatrists, psychologists, or social workers is limited across the country, but it is particularly critical in the rural areas. Fifty-five percent of all U.S. counties do not have access to a mental health specialist; of these, all of the underserved counties are rural (National Advisory Committee on Rural Health, 1993). The problems with access and availability of mental health care and social support services are particularly severe among rural minorities, who tend to be concentrated in resource poor communities.

Several programmatic policies have been implemented to address the inequities of health care availability between rural and urban areas. These include a change in designation of "psychiatric professional shortage areas" to "mental health professional shortage areas" (MHPSAs) to allow additional funds in rural areas for providers and other resources, continued (albeit limited) funding by the National Health Service Corps, and federally funded interdisciplinary training projects such as the Area Health Education Centers (AHECs). Despite these efforts, the disparities remain relatively unchanged. Interdisciplinary collaborations have begun to result in the deployment of nonphysician health care personnel such as nurse practitioners, psychologists, and social workers to improve access to health care services, but reimbursement for the services of these individuals and provision of prescription drug treatments is limited by the issue of credentialing. More effective policies are needed which address the recruitment and retention of physicians and other health professions to rural areas.

In Chapter 2, McNamara advances the concept that the creation of an interdisciplinary curriculum focused on the needs of rural women could lead to improved access to appropriately trained and sensitive health personnel for rural women. Efforts to improve linkages between mental, behavioral, and physical health, and the development of innovative service delivery models that encourage interventions around natural support networks, are also cited as strategies that might facilitate access.

McNamara also introduces the concept of "permanence" in rural practitioner availability and discusses a number of perspectives on this topic. Recruiting and retaining health care providers is but one aspect of the issue. McNamara postulates that efforts to attract rural residents into the health care workforce, as well as the continued development of rural training sites, need to be facilitated. Although the support of providers through telehealth initiatives and distance learning opportunities is becoming a reality, as discussed in chapter 13, whether the availability of information technology will increase the "permanence" of practitioners in rural areas is unclear at this time. Finally, the amount of information available to patients and practitioners on the Internet is expanding rapidly, and has incredible potential to support, expand, and improve the lives and health of rural residents, both men and women.

Federal and state regulations have a major impact on factors influencing "permanence." Removing financial disincentives to practice in rural areas, as well as establishing policies that promote integration of services, facilitate reimbursement and other funding supports, and stimulate collaborative practice among various levels of health care providers could positively influence the availability of practitioners in rural areas.

In Chapter 13, Jameson describes a successful collaboration among several hospitals in the state of Washington. A unique collaboration of five hospitals in the city of Spokane, known as Inland Northwest Health Services (INHS), utilized technology to demonstrate an effective strategy to meet rural health care and education needs. The initiative started as a collaborative effort between two competing hospitals that were faced with declining operating margins. The collaboration eventually became a single health delivery system that provides higher-quality and more efficient patient care. Northwest TeleHealth is one outgrowth of the collaborative efforts of INHS. The Northwest TeleHealth technology network is utilized to provide both telehealth services (communications and computer technologies utilized to transfer medical information and expertise for clinical, educational, research, and administrative applications) and telemedicine (specific application to patient care).

The various applications of telehealth and telemedicine technology that could be more broadly applied to rural populations are detailed in Chapter 13. The model described in the Spokane example might be applicable to other urban/rural settings for provision of direct services, consultation with specialists, health care provider support and education, and consumer education. One rapidly emerging use of telecommunication technology is in the area of home health care. The utilization of home monitoring equipment and telecommunications technology has allowed patients to receive follow-up care and monitoring in their homes. Such applications offer hope for isolated rural persons with serious chronic diseases such as congestive heart failure, diabetes, and depression.

Nevertheless, other barriers to expansion and greater incorporation of telehealth technologies exist. The financial cost of equipment and installation of transmission lines in rural areas is significant, and continued availability of federal support to initiate such systems is uncertain. The ability of telemedicine systems to maintain financial viability, once established, is also in question. Although states have different rules and restrictions with regard to the reimbursement of clinical services via telemedicine networks, the lack of reimbursement for direct specialist services, the lack of long-term funding sources, and questions about the acceptance of the use of telemedicine by traditional health care practitioners may limit the promise of this technology opportunity.

ARE RURAL WOMEN STRESSED?

In a fascinating study on the effects of race and poverty on perceived stress in rural women, detailed in Chapter 11, Probst, Moore, and Baxley found that although the stressors of low income, low education, and poor health status were more prevalent in rural areas and among minorities, the prevalence of perceived stress was slightly less among rural women than urban women. This effect held true across racial groups, despite the greater prevalence of chronic life difficulties in minority populations. Minority race was associated with a lower probability of reporting high stress. Rural Hispanic and African American women, who had significantly more life difficulties, were less likely to report high stress than were rural White women. Similarities of stress patterns occurred among all groups of women, urban and rural, minority and other, and with certain "critical" indicators such as recent serious personal or emotional problems, perceived poor health, and employment outside the home.

Further study is needed to explore the effects of urban and rural residence, race, and low income on experienced stress. The findings by Probst and colleagues indicate that despite the greater exposure to externally defined stressors such as low income, lower employment, and little or no health insurance, rural women—and particularly minority rural women—seem to experience less stress than their urban, White counterparts. Minority status seems to confer some protection from experiencing stress among African American and Hispanic women, both rural and urban. Future research into experienced stress might explore the unique sources of internal and external support in these groups and the sources of resilience found in rural residents and among certain minority groups, which have an impact on the internal perceptions of stress among individuals. The separation of stressors from stress suggests a future line of research to investigate the mental and physical attributes of resilience or hardiness, and how such strengths might be promoted in communities.

While all rural women face challenges that can contribute to mental health problems, older rural women in particular are at risk for increased depressive and anxiety symptoms. Chapter 3, by Gold, Dominick, Ahern, and Heller, summarizes previous research identifying problems of older rural women that can contribute to negative effects on their mental health. These include physical problems that may lead to depression, such as cardiac disease, diabetes, and health problems that lead to losses in functioning. Mental health problems that result from stress due to caregiving roles, isolation due to rural geography, disability (which contributes to isolation), and loneliness, often as a result of widowhood, are also cited.

In their study of more than 28,000 older women enrolled in an income-based pharmaceutical program in Pennsylvania, Gold and her coauthors found that although urban women reported more days of anxiety, rural women were more likely to be taking prescribed anxiolytics. They also found that whereas 20–25 percent of these women were taking anxiolytics during a 12-month period, only 3.7 percent had a physician's diagnosis code of anxiety during this time period. While there was no rural/urban difference in self-reported number of depressed mood days, rural women were less likely to have a diagnosis code of depression. Yet, despite the fewer codes for depression for rural women, they were as likely as urban women to fill prescriptions for antidepressant medication. As was the case with anxiolytics, only a very small percentage of rural and urban women (2.7 percent and 3.5 percent, respectively) had diagnosis codes for depression in the year during which approximately 17 percent were taking antidepressants.

Gold and colleagues expressed concern regarding this large number of both rural and urban women receiving prescriptions for psychotropic medications for which there was no diagnosis during the 12-month period of the study. It may be that the physicians diagnosing these medicated elderly are indeed monitoring their psychological disorders and the results reflect under-reporting of mental disorders. Nevertheless, these psychotropic drugs require surveillance because of potential adverse effects. This is especially true for the rural elderly, who may be alone for long periods of time. The authors also expressed concern that rural women on antidepressants were less likely to be receiving drugs in the category of selective serotonin reuptake inhibitors (SSRIs), compared with urban women. The SSRIs appear to be a safer choice of pharmacologic therapy for the geriatric population.

It is important that future research examine the reasons for these rural/urban differences in psychotropic medication use, as well as the lack of physician coding of the mental health conditions for which these medications have been prescribed. The knowledge gained from Gold's research may provide a foundation for better training of rural health care providers to ensure a higher quality of mental health assessment and treatment of older women.

OBESITY AND NUTRITION CONSIDERATIONS IN RURAL WOMEN

Obesity is a very common health and nutrition problem for women in both rural and urban environments. However, research from various databases indicates that rural White women tend to be about five pounds heavier than their urban counterparts. This pattern has been observed in the Northeast and South, but not in the Midwest and West. The reason for these geographical differences is not known. It is known, however, that there is an inverse relationship between socioeconomic status and education level, on the one hand, and obesity and overweight, on the other, in both rural and urban populations. Because socioeconomic status and educational attainment tend to be lower among rural women, this may partially explain the higher rates of obesity seen in rural areas.

Olson and Bove, in Chapter 4, considered the relationship of food insecurity to obesity, and also attempted to determine whether a disordered pattern of eating is related to food insecurity and obesity in a sample of rural women. They found that both food insecurity and a disordered pattern of eating are positively and independently associated with obesity. A multivariate analysis conducted by the authors revealed that women who lived in households characterized by food insecurity were almost twice as likely to be obese than women whose food source and availability were secure. Furthermore, women who had a disordered pattern of eating, particularly an eating pattern that included binges, were almost three times more likely to be obese. Mirroring the findings of other studies, higher education level was negatively associated with obesity, as was older age.

What are the sociocultural factors that may affect these findings? In an effort to deepen our understanding of the factors contributing to obesity in rural low-income women, Olson and Bove studied women in two rural communities from upstate New York. Using a qualitative approach, the preliminary data from this study, outlined in Chapter 4, seemed to confirm data from earlier qualitative research suggesting that physical activity, such as walking, is vital to women's weight management and that women who live in rural communities, where walking can be easily incorporated into daily activities, tend to have lower rates of obesity. On the other hand, women who are truly isolated, either because they live outside of rural population centers, or because of their own physical limitations, are at particular risk for obesity due to their sedentary lifestyles.

Parrett's research, presented in Chapter 12, describes a nutrition education and exercise health promotion program conducted with older adults living in a subsidized apartment facility. A strong body of evidence has demonstrated the importance of both nutritional well-being and exercise for reducing disease risk and better management of chronic diseases prevalent in older adults. Nutrition and exercise are important factors in maintaining both cognitive abilities and physical functions. Parrett reports on the efficacy of a program designed to promote both physical and mental health benefits for seniors, most of whom were White females living in housing communities. Four nutrition classes were provided during an eight-week period; both chair exercises and walking were encouraged. A significant finding for the well-being of rural older persons is that those who exercised more and who were at lower nutrition risk reported fewer depressive symptoms.

Studies such as these have limitations, including a small sample and no control group. However, the study participants are not unlike other rural older adults, with almost one quarter classified as high nutritional risk, with a high prevalence of overweight, and with about 10 percent classified with symptoms of depression. The study demonstrated that nutrition risk scores and timed-walk scores improved with a relatively modest and appropriate intervention provided in a readily accessible location. However, increases post intervention were attributed to the powerful effects of the September 11 terrorist attacks. Whether the improvements will last over time is yet to be determined.

In promoting a research agenda for the future, the study provides challenges for future program design and evaluation. What are accessible sites and delivery modes for most rural older adults? What are the best programs for adults who are at highest risk for physical and mental disabilities? Who should provide the programs and what is the cost/benefit ratio of effective interventions? These and other questions will await further study by these and other women's health researchers.

ACCESS TO MENTAL HEALTH SERVICES

A major theme, presented in different variations throughout the book, is the challenge to provide mental health services in rural communities. The interrelationship between mental and physical health, and between mental health and behavioral health are linked closely to the overall health of communities: In this regard, the health of rural America is "at risk." Finding solutions to the difficulty of providing mental health services for rural populations and preventing comorbidity, disability, and other consequences of mental illness, is a significant rural—and national—policy need.

The incidence of mental health problems is higher in females than in males. While evidence suggests that the prevalence of mental illness is similar in urban and rural areas, the number of providers is not, so that access to professional help for women living in rural areas is a significant concern.

What do we know about the utilization of mental health services among rural women? Previous studies have shown that depressed rural residents are more likely to negatively label those who seek professional treatment (Rost, Smith, & Taylor, 1993), suggesting that the stigma associated with mental illness, and possibly the lack of anonymity in rural communities, are barriers to accessing mental health services in the rural areas.

In Chapter 7, Shinogle describes the prominent features of rural women utilizing mental health services data from the 1996 and 1997 Medical Expenditure Panel Survey (MEPS), a nationally representative sample of the U.S. population gathered by the Agency for Healthcare Research Quality (AHRQ). The rural women represented in these data are more likely to be White (80 percent vs. 72 percent), married (58 percent vs. 54 percent), and slightly older (47 years vs. 45 years) than their urban counterparts. They are more likely to be in lower income categories and to be less educated than urban women. The data correlate strongly with access to health insurance coverage. Rural females are more likely than urban women to be uninsured. They may be ineligible for Medicaid, yet not have access to private health insurance coverage. These characteristics might explain a decreased utilization rate of health services among rural women, yet Shinogle did not find this to be the case. There was no difference in the percentage of rural women who utilized any mental health services compared with urban women. Further, there was no significant difference in the total mental health and substance abuse treatment expenditure by rural urban status.

An important finding in the study by Shinogle is the difference in service provision in the African American minority population. Controlling for age, poverty status, mental health status, and education level, rural African American women have significantly lower odds of receiving any mental health and/or substance abuse treatment than rural White women (56 percent vs. 68 percent). Is the difference due to a lack of providers or a lack of access to providers? Are there other forms of treatment, medical or nonmedical, that are being utilized for mental health and/or substance abuse treatment? The health disparities in rural minority populations (both male and female) represent an area that needs greater research attention.

The prevalence rate of psychiatric disorders does not appear to differ between urban and rural populations (Robins & Regier, 1991). Rural residents, however, and in particular rural women, use mental health services at a significantly lower rate than do women living in other areas. The Mental Health Parity Act, enacted by Congress in 1996, established new federal standards for mental health coverage offered under most employer-sponsored group health plans. However, the Mental Health Parity Act applies only to employer sponsored plans of 50 or more employees that fall under the umbrella of the Employee Retirement Income Security Act (ERISA). These restrictions may effectively preclude many working-age rural women with chronic mental illness from accessing mental health services, even if they are available in their small communities.

The results of research conducted by Olson and Bove at the Texas A&M School of Rural Public Health, and outlined in Chapter 4, were not surprising. Women with chronic mental illnesses living in rural areas have reduced work and lower wages compared with their urban counterparts, and are more likely not to have employment-based health insurance, even if they are working. The differences are more significant for rural African American and Hispanic women, and women living in the rural South and rural West. These vulnerable women, who often suffer from chronic mental illness, who are living and working in rural areas, and who are often employed on a parttime basis by small businesses with fewer than 50 employees, are effectively precluded from accessing the mental health coverage available through the Mental Health Parity Act. Such factors must be addressed as part of any comprehensive remedy to increase the availability and accessibility of mental health services in rural areas.

A number of financial barriers to the use of mental health services have been identified, including lack of ability to pay for services and the decreased likelihood of insurance plans that include coverage for mental health services. Government funding decisions may also impede the provision of mental health care services for rural residents, including women, since the public mental health system is often the only source of services for rural residents. The federally funded system of Community Mental Health Centers, later funded under the Mental Health Block Grant (OBRA), has seen restrictions and limitations in funding such that only persons with very severe mental illness are able to receive treatment. Those with less severe disorders or comorbid conditions of mental health disorder and substance abuse are least likely to be able to access services.

Many of the elderly, who have basic health insurance coverage for physical disease through the Medicare program, are not covered for mental health problems. Mental health benefits are available only through supplemental insurance purchased by the elderly Medicare recipient. The RUPRI Rural Health Panel found that only a small minority (16 percent) had access to Medicare + Choice plan in their area in 2001, compared with 82 percent of urban residents (Rural Policy Research Institute, 2003). Low-income elderly individuals who are financially eligible may have both Medicare and Medicaid coverage. While Medicaid pays for acute mental health services provided by mental health or primary care providers, the few providers located in rural areas may not be inclined to accept the lower rates of reimbursement provided by the Medicaid program.

Finally, there are barriers to accessing mental health services related to the disparities in health care providers, including mental health care providers, who are located in rural areas. A substantial portion of the mental health care in these areas is provided by primary-care physicians. These individuals may be overburdened by the general health needs of patients in their rural practice, be less trained in mental health problems, and have less support from community and social service agencies than that which is available in an urban environment.

Cultural barriers to accessing mental health services may include the stigma associated with having a mental health problem, negative labeling of those who receive treatment for mental health problems, and a sociocultural belief present in rural communities that mental health problems are best approached through the domains of church and family. A study by Gehlert, Kovac, Song, and Hartlage, discussed in Chapter 8, demonstrated that attitudes toward seeking mental health services were strongly associated with the utilization of mental health services. Rural women had less favorable attitudes toward seeking mental health services than other groups, which accounted, at least in part, for the high percentage of women who did not seek services. A fascinating finding from this study is that the distance from the provider was *negatively* correlated with likelihood of utilization of mental health services. The authors suggest that *distance* may actually be a variable indicating the perception of stigma.

Gehlert's findings suggest that public health initiatives aimed at changing attitudes might increase the rates of treatment among rural women with mental and substance abuse problems, even as the financial and fiscal barriers are being addressed through other mechanisms. These findings also warrant further study in different locales and among those of various ethnic groups to ensure that results can be generalized, and to determine the implications for further action.

SPECIFIC POPULATIONS

Chapter 10 by Goodwin, Williams, and Dilworth-Anderson helps us to understand the similarities and disparities between rural and urban African American women, and how they may affect depressive symptoms. The authors focus on the importance of personal, social, and economic resources in emotional health, and they summarize previous research findings regarding these resources among African American women. The authors point out that the isolation of rural life, and the more limited health resources in rural communities, may contribute to worse mental health among rural-dwelling African American women. Research conducted by the authors did not confirm this premise, however. In their study of African American female caregivers in North Carolina, Goodwin and colleagues found that rates of depressive symptoms did not differ between rural and urban African American women. They found some support for the importance of personal, social, and economic resources on the emotional health of both rural and urban African Americans. The exception, interestingly, was that church participation increased depressive symptoms.

Goodwin and colleagues found an important difference between rural and urban African American women: Good health was a stronger predictor of emotional health among African American rural women than among urban women. The authors postulate that poor health may be more of a burden in rural communities because of the fewer resources available for those with physical health problems, such as specialized transportation or support groups. Also, previous research findings noted that many African Americans only seek medical help when a crisis occurs, leaving many chronic health problems untreated. Goodwin and colleagues stress the importance of further research regarding the impact of poor physical health on the emotional health of rural African American women, as compared with urban African American women. Epidemiologic research might be utilized to examine the types and severity of physical health problems encountered by rural and urban African American women. Previous findings have shown that rural persons suffer from higher incidences of chronic illness and experience more morbidity related to diabetes, cancer, hypertension, heart disease, stroke, and lung disease than do urban persons. With the knowledge that severe chronic medical illness can lead to depression, it is important that future research examine the relationship between physical and emotional health among rural African American women. Only then can programs be designed to promote behavioral changes to lessen the burden of illness on both the physical and mental health of African American women.

Racial and Ethnic Approaches to Community Health (REACH 2010) is part of the U.S. Department of Health and Human Services response to President Clinton's initiative to eliminate by 2010 disparities in health status experienced by racial and ethnic minorities in the priority areas of infant mortality, breast and cervical cancer, cardiovascular disease, diabetes, HIV infections and AIDS, and child and adult immunizations. The Oklahoma REACH 2010 Coalition was formed in 1999. It focuses efforts on reducing cardiovascular disease, diabetes, and their risk factors among American Indians in Oklahoma through increased availability and promotion of physical activity on a community level.

The goal of a research project conducted by Campbell et al. described in Chapter 9, was to assess the health status of rural American Indian women living in Oklahoma regarding several chronic conditions, their major risk factors, and health care access and use. Data for the project were accumulated from the Oklahoma REACH 2010 Behavioral Risk Factor Surveillance Survey (BRFSS) and the Oklahoma BRFSS. Data from female respondents were included in the study and were classified as either urban or rural. Rural American Indian women in Oklahoma were compared to non-American Indian or Alaska Native women in Oklahoma.

The authors found that rural American Indian women in Oklahoma were at increased risk of daily cigarette smoking. The risk of diseases associated with cigarette smoking, such as COPD, asthma, coronary heart disease, and cancers such as lung, mouth, larynx, bladder, cervix, uterus, and pancreas was higher among rural American Indian women in Oklahoma compared with non-American Indian/ Alaska Native Oklahoma women.

Rural American Indian women in Oklahoma have an increased prevalence of overweight and obesity compared with non-American Indian/Alaska Native Oklahoma women and were at an increased risk for disorders related to overweight and obesity. These women were also disproportionately affected by a high prevalence of diabetes. There were no significant differences in the prevalence of heart disease or myocardial infarction or stroke. However, rural American Indian women may be at an increased risk of dying from these conditions and thus show lower rates of prevalence. Of note, rural American Indian women were significantly more likely to participate in physical activity or exercise than non-American Indian/Alaska Native women.

Rural American Indian women have higher rates of health insurance coverage due to the availability of services through the Indian Health Services and the Tribal Health Services, but these services are underutilized and are not comprehensive. Thus, almost one in five rural American Indian women need medical care but are unable to get it because of cost.

Rural American Indian women have poor physical or mental health that keeps them from doing their usual activities for 11.3 days per month, compared with 4.5 days per month among non-American Indian/Alaska Native Oklahoma women. One in four rural American Indian women reported that they have limitations because of health impairment, compared with 18.1 percent of non-American Indian/ Alaska Native Oklahoma women.

The authors conclude that while decreasing risk factors should be the primary purpose of prevention programs, these programs will be successful only if they are planned and implemented by the community in conjunction with the funding source. Targeted programs will have to be designed that take into account the characteristics of the community, including demographics, specific risk patterns and incidence of chronic disease, as well as the prevailing attitude of the community toward prevention and risk modification.

In Chapter 5, Hillemeier, Weisman, and colleagues describe a research project aimed at rural women of reproductive age. The Central Pennsylvania Women's Health Study (CEPAWHS) Project has two main objectives: (1) to obtain comprehensive information on the health status of rural women, and (2) to promote the health of high-risk rural women prior to pregnancy through a multidimensional intervention. The project will conduct a population-based survey of reproductive-age women in a 28-county region in Central Pennsylvania that includes a large rural population. The survey will collect data to determine the prevalence of risk factors for preterm birth and low birthweight and the relationships among risk factors and race/ethnicity, socioeconomic status, rural residence, and women's health care access and utilization patterns. Topics will include pregnancy history, health status, psychosocial stress, health behaviors, health care access and utilization, and sociodemographics. Once the information is obtained, an intervention will be designed that will target the prevalent risk factors in women who are not yet pregnant. The goal of the intervention is to reduce preterm birth and low birthweight among rural women through reduction of health risks prior to pregnancy.

RECOMMENDATIONS FOR FUTURE RESEARCH

Throughout this chapter, we have identified a number of areas that warrant additional research, particularly those that relate to the research projects described in each individual chapter of the book. Rural women's health is a relatively new focus of attention in the research arena. The entire arena of women's health has only recently received recognition as the National Institutes of Health (NIH) Office of Women's Health Research was created and the field of sex-based biology emerged. First, there is a need to further define the differences in health—physical and mental—found in the populations of women related to their residential demographic (rural vs. urban). Although some of this epidemiologic research has been compiled and presented in this book, additional research needs to be done.

Many of the studies detailed in this book note discrepancies in the research demographic termed "rural." As future research is undertaken, there is a clear need to further define "rural," and to standardize the definitions of this and related terms including semi-rural, semiurban, nonurban, metropolitan, nonmetropolitan, etc. In addition, vigorous research needs to be done to enhance existing databases and to develop new data sets that reflect the more refined rural categories. Once demographic differences have been more completely described through additional research, a much deeper analysis of the variables causing these differences can be accomplished. The result will be a greater understanding of the impact of rural status on health and disease in women.

There is a significant need to expand epidemiologic research related to defining and understanding ethnic and cultural differences, regardless of geographical location. Further, additional research is needed to evaluate ethnic and cultural differences among women as they relate to location (i.e., rural vs. urban). How are the health disparities that exist between ethnic groups affected by place of residence? Why do rural women suffer higher rates of chronic illness and greater morbidity from chronic diseases?

Further study needs to be undertaken to understand the effects of urban and rural residence, race, and economic status on experienced stress. Separation of the concept of stressors (external stimuli) from "stress" as a personal, internal perception, will be important in future research to identify and investigate sources of resilience, hardiness, and emotional strength.

The further delineation and description of the behavioral factors that provide strength and support to rural women may provide information that might help rural women in their communities. Such factors, which positively affect a woman's physical and emotional well being, are being identified under the topic of resiliency. Identifying the factors which contribute to resiliency—factors such as close relationships, strong ties to extended family, and spiritual wellness—may provide rural women with strategies and mechanisms to better manage the multiple stressors and challenges of rural life.

Mental health research needs to expand its boundaries in order to focus on rural women. The multitude of issues that affect the mental health of rural women is both similar to and different from that of urban women, but solutions to the problems of access, availability of mental health care, availability of specialty services, community support services, and financing of mental health care services will be distinctly rural in their design.

There is a clear need for outcomes-based research which would evaluate the efficacy of rural implementation of social programs and interventions designed for use in more urban settings. The inclusion of individuals living in rural areas in clinical research is important and problematic. Are the results of clinical trials applicable regardless of residential environment? How can research on rural-specific issues such as environmental exposure and traumatic injury be promoted? What applications of telehealth and telemedicine technology will result in greater access to services and improved health outcomes? What are accessible sites and delivery modes for programs and studies of rural populations?

Additional efforts need to be devoted to the factors necessary to attract, support, and retain health care service providers. Training experiences in the rural environment, and training curricula which will prepare practitioners for rural practice are needed, along with federal policies which address manpower shortages and geographical maldistribution (some of these policies already exist but need to be strengthened). Study of services provided by nonphysician health care professionals (nurse practitioners, nurse midwives, physician assistants) needs to be undertaken in order to influence policymaking.

The impact of computers and Internet access to health education and resources needs to be studied to determine the impact on the risk status and health of various populations, including rural women. As technology advances into the schools, libraries, and homes of rural residents, the connection to information and resources may improve the lives and health of those in otherwise isolated rural environments.

Finally, the current focus on health disparities research needs to be expanded to include the differences in health and disease experienced by rural and urban residents, both male and female, as well as the existing definition of health disparities, which identifies health differences between various ethnic populations.

REFERENCES

Arizona Health Care Cost Containment System (2001). Initiatives to Improve Access to Rural Health Care Services, A Briefing Paper. Retrieved October 8, 2004, from http://www.ahcccs.state.az.us/Studies/HRSAGrant/RuralPaper.pdf

Casey, M. M., Call, K. T., & Klingner, J. M. (2001). Are rural residents less likely to obtain recommended preventive healthcare services? *American Journal of Preventive Medicine 21*(3), 182–188.

Centers for Disease Control and Prevention (1997). Atlas reveals new mortality patterns for the United States. Available at http://www.cdc.gov/od/oc/media/presserel/deaths.htm.

Duelberg, S. I. (1992). Preventive health behavior among Black and White women in urban and rural areas. *Social Sciences Medicine, 34*(2), 191–198.

Health Resources and Services Administration (2003). *The Quentin N. Burdick Rural Program for Interdisciplinary Training.* Retrieved September 10, 2003, from http://bhpr.hrsa.gov/shortage.

Larson, E. H., Hart, L. G., & Rosenblatt, R. A. (1997). Is nonmetropolitan residence a risk factor for poor birth outcome in the U.S.? *Social Science and Medicine, 45*(2), 171–188.

Lishner, D. M., Larson, E. H., Rosenblatt, R. A., & Clark, S. J. (1999). Rural maternal and perinatal health. In T. C. Ricketts (Ed.), *Rural health in the United States.* New York: Oxford University Press.

National Advisory Committee on Rural Health (1993). *Sixth annual report on rural health.* Rockville, MD: U.S. Department of Health and Human Services.

Peck J., & Alexander K. (2003). Maternal, infant, and child health in rural areas: A literature review. In L. D. Gamm, L. Hutchison, B. J. Dabney, & A. M. Dorsey, *Rural Health People 2010: A companion document to Healthy People 2010*, Vol. 2. College Station, TX: Texas A&M University System Health Science Center.

Robins, L. N., & Regier, D. A. (1991). *Psychiatric disorders in America: The Epidemiologic Catchment Area study.* New York: Free Press.

Rost, K., Smith, G. R., & Taylor, J. L. (1993). Rural-urban differences in stigma and the use of care for depressive disorders. *Journal of Rural Health, 9*(1), 57–62.

Rural Policy Research Institute (2003). *Inequitable access: Medicare + Choice program fails to serve rural America.* Retrieved August 22, 2003, from http://www.rupri.org/ruralhealth/publications/PB2003-5.pdf

U.S. Department of Agriculture (2000). Rural Income, Poverty, and Welfare: Rural Poverty. Available at http://www.ers.usda.gov.briefing/IncomePovertyWelfar/ruralpoverty/

U.S. Department of Agriculture (1998). *Metro and nonmetro income data based on census information.* Available at http://www.usda.gov.news/pubs/fbook98/ch4e.htm

U.S. Department of Agriculture (1997). *Census of agriculture.* Washington, DC: U.S. Government Printing Office.

Author Index

Subject Index

SPRINGER / PUBLISHING COMPANY

Rural Nursing, *2nd Edition*
Concepts, Theory, and Practice

Helen J. Lee, PhD, RN
Charlene A. Winters, DNSc, APRN, BC, Editors

This thoroughly revised second edition chronicles the path to creating a coherent, conceptual framework for rural nursing practice. By bringing together research, theory, and narratives from rural nursing practice, the authors and contributors provide readers with a foundation for understanding the special dimensions of rural nursing and health, including:

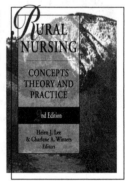

• The need for nurses to play multiple autonomous and team-centered roles
• Negotiating issues of confidentiality and over-familiarity with the lives of patients
• Self-reliant rural dwellers often seeking healthcare as a last resort
• Life-or-death roles that remote locations often play in whether health care is accessed in a timely manner
• Environmental health hazards due to hazardous waste in rural areas

Partial Contents:

Part I: The Rural Nursing Theory Base • Rural Nursing • Re-examining the Rural Theory Base • Exploring Rural Nursing Theory Across Borders

Part II: Perspectives of Rural Persons • Health Needs and Perceptions of Rural Persons • Health Perceptions, Needs, and Behaviors of Remote Rural Women of Childbearing and Child Rearing Age • Strategizing Safety • Rural Family Health

Part III: The Rural Dweller and Response to Illness • Patterns of Responses to Symptoms in Rural Residents • Updating the Symptom-Action-Time-Line • The Chronic Illness Experience

Part IV: Rural Nursing Practice • The Distinctive Nature and Scope of Rural Nursing Practice • Rural Health Professionals' Perceptions of Lack of Anonymity • Rural Nurse Generalist in Community Health • Men Working as Rural Nurses • Continuing Education and Rural Nurses

Part V: Rural Public Health • Public Health Emergency Preparedness in Rural/Frontier Areas • Rural School Health • Improving the Health Literacy of Rural Elders

Part VI : Looking Ahead • Further Development of the Rural Nursing Theory Base • Implications for Education, Practice, and Policy

November 2005   384pp   0-8261-6955-4   softcover

11 West 42nd Street, New York, NY 10036-8002 • Fax: 212-941-7842
Order Toll-Free: 877-687-7476 • Order On-line: www.springerpub.com